D1154806

CARING
CURING
COPING

CARING   *Nurse*

CURING   *Physician*

COPING   *Patient*

Relationships

edited by   *Anne H. Bishop*

and

John R. Scudder, Jr.

The University of Alabama Press

6-28-94

Library of Congress Cataloging in Publication Data

Main entry under title:

Caring, curing, coping.

Papers presented at the Conference "Coping, Curing,
Caring: Patient, Physician, Nurse Relationships,"
held Apr. 8–9, 1983, in Lynchburg, Va., and sponsored by
the Depts. of Philosophy and Nursing at Lynchburg
College.
Bibliography: p.
Includes index.
1. Nursing ethics—Congresses.   2. Nurse and
physician—Congresses.   3. Nurse and patient—Congresses.
4. Interpersonal relations—Congresses.   I. Bishop,
Anne H., 1935– .   II. Scudder, John R., 1926– .
III. Conference "Coping, Curing, Caring: Patient,
Physician, Nurse Relationships" (1983 : Lynchburg, Va.)
IV. Lynchburg College Dept. of Philosophy.
V. Lynchburg College. Dept. of Nursing.   [DNLM:
1. Ethics, Medical—congresses.   2. Ethics, Nursing—
congresses.   3. Interprofessional Relations—congresses.
4. Nurse-Patient Relations—congresses.   5. Physician-
Patient Relations—congresses. W 62 C276 1983]
RT85.C28 1985   610.73'06'99   84-8836
ISBN 0-8173-0242-5

Contents

Acknowledgments

This publication was made possible by a grant from the Virginia Foundation for the Humanities and Public Policy. We acknowledge with gratitude the material support of the Foundation and, in particular, we wish to thank Robert Vaughan, the Executive Director of the Foundation, and his staff for their suggestions, encouragement, and support. By partially funding this publication, the Foundation makes possible the wider consideration of a neglected theme in philosophy and medicine that was treated at a conference the Foundation supported. The Conference, "Coping, Curing, Caring: Patient, Physician, Nurse Relationships," was sponsored by the Departments of Philosophy and Nursing at Lynchburg College, Lynchburg, Virginia, and funded through a grant from the Virginia Foundation for the Humanities and Public Policy. We appreciate the support of the College and the Foundation in making the Conference a reality.

In addition to the papers of the five major speakers at the Conference, participants used a film and case studies to discuss the implications of relationships between patients, physicians, and nurses. We thank our Colleagues in the Departments of Philosophy and Nursing at Lynchburg College for leading the discussions. Appreciation is also extended to the many nursing students at the College who assisted with registration and served as group observers.

The extra time and effort that goes into any project is usually made possible by the support of caring persons who often go unnoticed. In the case of this Conference

Acknowledgments

and book, Mary and Bobby, our spouses, gave us such support. Ernestine Dodl, Secretary to the Department of Nursing, made contributions far beyond duties normally associated with her work.

Edmund D. Pellegrino's article includes material from his previous article "'The Common Devotion'—Cushing's Legacy and Medical Ethics Today," *Journal of Neurosurgery* 59 (1983): 567–73, and Sally A. Gadow's article includes her previous article "Touch and Technology: Two Paradigms of Patient Care," *Journal of Religion and Health* 23 (1): 63–69. Both are used with permission of the editors and publishers. The extensive quotations from Robert C. Hardy's *Sick* (Chicago: Teach 'em, Inc., 1978) included in Richard M. Zaner's article are used with permission of the editor and publisher.

CARING
CURING
COPING

Introduction

Recent advances in medical tech-
nology and science have brought bioethical issues to the
forefront of medical and philosophical literature. These
issues concern such areas as death and dying, informed
consent, abortion, genetic manipulation, contraception
and sterilization, artificial insemination, and euthanasia.
The usual approach to these issues is to point out that
medical science and technology have made it possible for
us to intervene in the life processes in ways that human
beings previously have not been capable of doing. As a
consequence of these interventions, medical practitioners are faced with new moral problems and dilemmas. To help resolve these issues, medical practitioners
are increasingly turning to humanists, and especially
philosophers. Philosophers use their expertise to clarify
the moral issues and to apply traditional, recognized
moral norms to contribute to their resolution. Thus medical practitioners learn to consider these moral dilemmas
in terms of the moral imperatives of happiness, duty,
utilitarianism, and I-Thou relationships. Doubtless, such

treatments are of considerable value to health practitioners.

Unfortunately, the bioethical approach has limitations. First, this approach focuses on the "big issues" of life support and life prolongation rather than on the everyday practice of health professionals, where most moral decisions are made. Second, bringing philosophical methodology and norms to bear on the problems removes the moral decision making further from the actual situation. Third, decision making, in a situation, involves many people other than those who have the medical and philosophical understanding necessary to resolve bioethical issues. Finally but foremost, the bioethical approach inadvertently implies that medical practice is basically an adjunct of science and technology.

The "big issues" in health care are not only of concern to health practitioners, but to the general public as well. For example, the issue of euthanasia was dramatically presented to the public by the media in the Karen Ann Quinlan case and in the movie *Whose Life Is It Anyway?* However, for all the attention given to the "big issues," only minimal consideration has been given to the moral issues involved in day-to-day health care and to the ongoing relationships of physicians, nurses, and patients. For example, a man is informed, after a routine physical examination, that he has a small hernia. He is advised by his physician to have it treated surgically as soon as possible and he follows the physician's expert advice. No consideration is given to the cost, to the danger, to the alternatives to surgery, or to other persons involved at home or work. In short, the only factors considered are medical, as prescribed by the physician and submitted to by the patient.

Or consider the case of an elderly female patient who is suffering from nagging, persistent pain. Her physician, believing the pain is not an indication of a serious medical problem but due to a chronic problem he believes is related to her age, delays seeing the patient for a month, due to his crowded schedule. This decision is made without considering the patient's suffering over the month, her anxiety whether the pain may be an indication of a more serious problem—that it may, in fact, be a symptom. This decision is made from the perspective of the physician's practice, without consideration of the physiological and psychological well-being of the woman over the next month.

Another example of not dealing with moral decisions in everyday situations is physicians' allowing receptionists to decide when patients will be examined.

It is difficult to imagine how one would treat these issues on a hedonistic, as opposed to a duty, norm. Further, it seems unlikely that most physicians and patients would be able to discuss moral issues in such a way. If they were capable of making medical decisions philosophically, would their time be well spent in constructing such philosophical analyses? Where would the physician find time to make ethical analyses of each case in his busy schedule?

No doubt, increased ability to formulate moral issues and think in terms of moral imperatives would help physicians set policy and deal with cases that involve exceptional moral issues. Our point is simply that most moral questions in medical practice in everyday care are faced with the limitations of time and philosophical abilities inherent in these situations.

The bioethical approach, which focuses on large issues, ignores the fact that at the everyday level of moral decisions many individuals are affected by a single decision. The patient, the family, the nurse, and other health workers—as well as the physician—should be involved in making decisions concerning the patient's health care. Moreover, the nature of this involvement depends on the situation. Is the patient competent to make his or her own decision? If so, is the patient financially responsible? What effect will this decision have on the patient's work and family?

For example, a family that had struggled long and hard to put the husband and father through graduate school plans an extended vacation as a celebration—just as a member of this family is advised to have elective surgery. Should the family be involved in the considerations? Or consider the case of a physician who prescribes a detailed procedure which requires a large amount of a nurse's time, and bends the institutional policy, without consulting the nurse. Does the physician have the right to dictate the nurse's schedule and to involve her in possible violation of institutional procedure without her consent?

The fourth limitation, the implications of the bioethical approach for medical practice, became evident to us through participating in our conference (April 8–9, 1983) and pondering the effects as editors of the proceedings. Actually, concern about the three limitations of the bioethical approach (discussed above) motivated our formulation and direction of the conference. We titled our conference "Coping, Curing, Caring: Patient, Physician, Nurse Relationships," with the expectation that in these relationships the patients were concerned primarily with coping, the physicians with curing, and the nurses with caring. These expectations are evident in the following quotation from the conference rationale:

The physician brings knowledge and skill regarding cure; the nurse brings knowledge and skill in caring; and the patient brings his values and concerns for a good and healthy life. Logically, any consideration of philosophical

Introduction

issues, and especially ethical ones, should focus on the relationship of curing and caring. The patient establishes a relationship with the physician or health care worker in order to cope with problems, situations, and changes in his way of being brought about as a result of illness.

This implies that caring, curing, and coping are related and interact with each other. In fact, we hoped that the conference would point to the necessity of patient, physician, and nurse working together to promote this interaction.

The speakers at the conference, as is evident in the following papers, regard the roles of both physician and nurse to be that of caring. Further, they hold that it is very difficult to draw a clear distinction between the roles of physician and nurse. Also, they contend that the stress on the scientific and technical side of health care, related to curing, threatens to move physicians and nurses away from their traditional caring relationship with patients.

After we examine the above considerations, it is possible to treat the fourth limitation of the bioethical approach, which implies that health care's primary function is curing. Its rationale is that advances in medical science require us to be concerned with moral issues in medicine. The assumption of our conference, and the following papers, is that the primary moral issues have been there all along in the relationship of health care workers and the patient.

The issues raised in bioethics give a certain urgency to the treatment of specific medical-moral issues. The interest in medical ethics generated by these new concerns can have one of two effects. It can convince us that the big, spectacular new issues are issues of moral importance, and thus blind us to the moral questions in everyday health care and to the relationships which underlie even the big issues, or it can focus our attention on the moral questions in the relationships of patients, physicians, nurses, and other health care workers. Certainly, many health care professionals have elected the second alternative. To them, biomedical ethics means making ethical judgments concerning moral issues that arise in actual practice. Further, it implies seeking the help of ethicists in making moral decisions. Thus biomedical ethics in practice does not necessarily mean what the name implies. Nevertheless, the term "biomedical ethics" implies that moral problems result primarily from applying science, especially biology, to medicine.

The moral issues that are treated by bioethicists often result from the tremendous strides made by applying science and technology to medicine. These issues are typically treated by applying the traditional procedures and norms of philosophical ethics to these problems. This cross-fertilization between medicine and philosophy has certainly been productive in dealing with moral issues that arise from medical practice. However, treating occasional moral problems as they arise in health care, especially when they result from the application of science to medicine, can lead to missing the primary thrust of medical ethics. After all, health care itself is a moral undertaking, in that its aim is the patient's well-being. The nature of this well-being and how it is to be attained are the primary concerns of medical ethics.

The following papers all focus on care for the patient's well-being—what this care means, how it is brought into being, and especially the relationships it requires. Thus all the contributors approach medical ethics from within health care practice, focusing on the moral imperative to care for the patient's well-being.

The caring ethic and the bioethic are rooted in different interpretations of health care. The bioethic focuses on the

Introduction

scientific and technological methods which made curing possible. In this interpretation of health care, the primary function of the physician is to cure and that of the nurse is to assist the physician in bringing about cure. The patient is considered an "illness" to be cured.

In contrast, the caring approach considers the patient a person who comes to the physician and nurse because his or her illness requires professional care. Cure, when possible, is an essential part of that care. But care requires cure in a way that is acceptable to the patient. Such care is not ultimately rooted in professional roles or medical science and technology, but in a relationship of mutual concern, respect, and support of persons for each other.

Edmund D.   **1. The Caring Ethic:**

Pellegrino   **The Relation of**

Physician to Patient

This symposium deals with the most fundamental topic in medical ethics today: the relationship between the person who is ill and those who profess to heal him—physicians, nurses, the family, the minister, and the social worker. My assignment is to focus on the ethical aspects of this relationship which have become so complicated in recent decades. I will base my comments not so much on the application of specific ethical principles regarding the rights of patients or the duties of health professionals. Rather, I will focus on the humane aspects of what it is to be ill and what it is to be healed. I want, in short, to concentrate more on the caring than the curing aspects of the relationship, and on the moral obligations subsumed in the notion of caring.

I make this distinction because in those two words, *cure* and *care*, the recent history of medicine is capsulized. The dominant notion in medicine for most of its history has been caring, even when the physician may have thought he was curing. It is only with the introduction of truly scientific means of therapeutics that cure has become possible in any real sense. As a result, the caring aspects of the healing relationship have come to be neglected, and even denigrated.

What is the relationship between caring and curing? What are the moral obligations of healers—physicians, nurses, all who come into direct hands-on contact with sick people?

It is interesting to note at the outset that both words, *curing* and *caring*, have the same Latin root: *curo, curare*— "to cure," "to take care of," " to take trouble," and later "to treat" medically and surgically, to "heal" or "restore" to health. For the greater part of medical history these various senses of curing and caring were essentially one. It is only with the beginnings of truly scientific and therapeutically effective, discrete therapies that the possibility of cure without care has existed.

The word *cure* is now used by many health professionals in a radical sense: to refer to the eradication of the cause of an illness or disease—to the radical interruption, and reversal, of the natural history of a disorder. The result of a "cure" is to restore a patient to at least the state he or she was in before the onset of illness and, possibly, to an even better state of functioning. The possibility of "cure," in this sense, turns on the availability of scientific medicine: truly effective therapeutic modalities which make it possible to cure without caring.

Specific, radical, and effective cures—in the technical sense—have been acquired in greatest profusion during the lifetime of physicians who entered the profession following World War II. Here and there, largely through empirical good fortune, some truly effective cures existed before that time (cinchona bark for malaria, foxglove for heart failure, mercury for syphilis), and some were discovered by scientific investigation earlier in this century (insulin, liver extract, sulfonamides). But the golden era of specific therapy has just begun, and its promises are still to be fully apprehended.[1] We are now in the era of synthesis of natural and man-made agents, designed to attack the molecular and cellular sources of disease. We can invade any body cavity to excise, reconstruct, or transplant diseased organs and tissues. Radical cure and restoration—not amelioration or disease containment—have become realistic and legitimate goals of medicine.

It is easy, and perhaps some think it desirable, to forget that the greatest part of the history of medicine was based in a different conception of cure, associated with care of the ill and sick. To be sure, the extensive pharmacopoeias of the Chinese, Indian, and Roman physicians implied curative powers. Fortuitously, some items in them *did* cure; but most were worthless or even dangerous. Cure, if it occurred, resulted largely from the body's self-healing powers and the physician's compassion, caring, encouragement, and emotional support.

The ancient grounding of medicine in care and compassion is now challenged by a biomedical model which defines medicine simply as applied biology.[2] On this approach, the primary function of medicine is to cure, and this requires that the physician be primarily a scientist. This model still includes containment of illness, by slowing down its progress and amelioration of its symptoms, but it focuses on *things* to do for a particular disease that are measurably effective.

In response to this narrow definition, some advocate a broader approach that adds the sociological and psychological aspects of illness.[3] Others would expand this further to a "holistic" approach, adding the religious and spiritual dimensions of illness to the bio-psycho-social model. These expanded concepts of medicine are limited by the impossibility that all physicians can acquire the requisite understandings and sensitivities the biopsychosocial model demands. Also, such a model tends to absorb all the health professions into medicine, expanding its pretensions beyond all reasonable hope of fulfillment.

In this essay, I wish to examine what we mean by "caring" and the necessity of a clear concept of the totality of its meaning as a basis for a reformulation of professional ethics. I will concentrate on professional medical ethics, largely to avoid the presumption, not unknown to physicians, of prescribing for other health professionals. I believe, however, that we are all joined in a common task of healing, helping, and caring and that the same moral obligations bind us all in those endeavors.

There are at least four senses in which the word *care* can be understood in the health professions.

The first sense is care as compassion—being concerned for another person; feeling or sharing something of his or her experience of illness and pain; being touched by the plight of another person. To care in this sense is to see the person who is ill, and at the center of our ministrations, as more than the object of our ministrations: as a fellow human whose experiences we cannot penetrate fully but which we can be touched by because we share the same humanity.

The second sense of caring is doing for others what they cannot do for themselves. This entails assisting them with all the activity of daily living that is compromised by illness: feeding, bathing, clothing, meeting personal needs—physical, social, and emotional. Physicians do little or none of this kind of care. Nurses do much more, but far less than they used to do. The large part of this kind of care is given by nurses' aides in today's "team nursing."

The third sense of caring is to take care of the medical

problem—to invite the patient to transfer responsibility and anxiety about what is wrong, and what can and should be done to the physician or nurse. This implies assurance that the latter will direct all appropriate knowledge and skill to the "problem" the patient presents, to intervene in the natural history of the disease.

The fourth sense of caring is to "take care": to carry out all the necessary procedures, personal and technical, with conscientious attention to detail, with perfection. This is a corollary of the third sense of care, but its emphasis is on the craftsmanship of medicine. Together, the third and fourth senses are what most physicians subsume under the rubric of *competence*.

These four senses of care are not separable in optimal clinical practice. Nonetheless, in reality, they are often separated, and even placed in opposition to each other. Or all four senses are reduced to one, to the exclusion of each.

For example, the biomedical model of the physician-patient relationship places emphasis on technical competence and conscientiousness, relegating the first two senses—which are more affective than technical—to other health professionals. On the other hand, the expansionist models of medicine—the holistic or biopsychosocial—embrace all dimensions of care, blurring the distinctions between them. Partitioning or conflating the four senses of care poses dangers to patients, because it either neglects one aspect or presumes to do too much.

It is essential that each sense of caring be recognized for its contribution to the healing relationship. Each must be placed in its proper place in an order of priorities determined by the needs of a particular patient. Care is of one piece. The challenge to health professionals is to attend to each sense of care, and thus relate one to the other, so that they enhance the healing relationship for each patient.

The Caring Ethic

In the ideal healing relationship (patient-physician, patient-nurse), each health professional would attend to each dimension of care in every ministration. When this is not possible, as in contemporary care, the four senses of caring must be provided by conscious partitioning of functions among members of the medical or health care team. The moment we make such divisions, we must appreciate that the unity of care is threatened. Special attention must then be exerted so that no aspect of caring is neglected, because no member of the health care team accepts the responsibility or sees it as proper to his or her professional tasks or status.

Integral care—that is to say, care that satisfies the four senses I have defined—is a moral obligation of health professionals. It is not an option they can exercise and interpret in terms of some idiosyncratic definition of professional responsibility. The moral obligation arises out of the special human relationship that binds one who is ill to one who offers to help.

To assess whether the curing or caring model is foundational for medical practice, it is necessary to examine the three fundamental elements of the physician-patient relationship.[4] The first element is the person who is ill and needs and seeks help. The second element is the act of profession—the promise the healer makes when he or she enters into the relationship with the person who is ill. The third element is the act of medicine or the act of healing. The following discussion of these three elements should make it clear that although curing and caring are essential parts of medical practice, caring "founds" that practice.

What is the meaning of being ill? Most people regard themselves as in a state of health, but this state cannot be determined absolutely. Despite all recent attempts to define health, no better functional definition has been given than by Galen, who defined health as that state in which we feel able to do the things we wish to do with minimum pain and discomfort. This means that you can feel you are in a state of health, and not feel ill, even though you have a disease. Indeed, many of us have disease within us, yet are able to do the things we want to do with minimum discomfort and disability. When something happens that shakes us out of this feeling of being in a healthy balance, it prompts us to seek help.

That balance is upset by a symptom: a pain in the chest, finding a lump, loss of appetite, morning nausea, dizziness on bending over—you name it. When such symptoms are perceived as a change in the function of our whole organism, they become sufficient to lead us to seek help. We become *patients* when we need help bearing a problem, a pain, a concern, an anxiety. It makes no difference whether a problem is emotional or physical; when we seek professional help, we become patients, and in becoming patients we enter a new existential state, of dependency and vulnerability. In this state, called *illness,* the body becomes the center of our concern because it is an impediment to, rather than a willing instrument for, the things we want to do.

The second element in the patient-physician relationship is the act of profession. When a patient enters a physician's office, the physician will say "What can I do for you?" or "How can I help you?" This is an act of profession, rather than a greeting, because within our social structure the physician is "ordained" as the one to whom the ill come for help. The physician's offer to help contains two implicit promises. First, the physician is competent and possesses the knowledge you need; second, he or she promises to use that knowledge in your interest.

The relationship of a vulnerable human (in the state of

illness) with another human who has declared and professed that he or she is competent to heal is different from a commercial or legal relationship. A commercial relationship is based on mutual self-interest; a legal relationship is based on contract. A patient-physician relationship is based on profession and trust. Patients must trust the physician because illness has disabled them, has forced them to face the fragility of personal existence and placed them in a vulnerable state where they are dependent on another human being. This extreme vulnerability requires that the physician's relationship to the patient be based not on mutual self-interest, or contract, but on profession.

The gap between the patient's illness and the physician's profession is closed in the act of medicine, the third element. This moment of clinical truth is the decision on what to do. Medicine does not come into existence until a decision is made about a particular human being in a particular life-context, here and now. Medicine, science, the biological sciences are preparatory for the moment of clinical truth, in which the physician and patient, together, decide what ought to be done.

What ought to be done has two elements: the *right* decision and the *good* decision. By "right" decision I mean that it must be technically correct, must use the best scientific knowledge. Therefore science is fundamental to all kinds of medicine. Medical science can determine what is physically wrong, what can be done about it, and what is likely to be the outcome; but it cannot tell what ought to be done for the *good* of a particular patient. If you follow the cure model, the biomedical model, then what is medically good—what is medically indicated, what is scientifically correct—becomes what is good for the patient.

But reflect for a moment and you'll see that the two are not the same. The good decision must also fit the particular person's concept of the good life and the way he or she wants to live. The good decision must fit the patient's value systems, belief systems, and (if present) religious and spiritual convictions. In short, a good decision, to the extent that is humanly possible, must take into account how the scientifically indicated fits into the particular values, beliefs, and convictions which define the patient as person.

All physicians face the conflict between a technically right curing decision and the patient's conception of the good decision. For example, this conflict often arises in treatment of a Jehovah's Witness, who can be cured of certain acute situations with a blood transfusion; but the Jehovah's Witness has religious convictions which, for him or her, preclude that possibility. The right decision technically is not the good decision, because it violates the promise that the physician will use his competence for the good of the person who is ill and vulnerable. A person in a vulnerable state is in an unequal relationship, in which another has control of his or her life at that moment. Obligations are greatest on the one who has this power in the healing relationship, because he or she has voluntarily professed to work for the good of this particular patient.

Cure, in the radical sense, is not the only aim of medicine. The end of medicine, in the philosophical sense, is a right and good healing decision for a particular human being. A medically right decision might be to resuscitate a critically ill patient in hope that time would eventually lead to cure. Or if a patient had said no ("I'm not willing to pay the price of continuing to suffer; I am ready to face death; I am ready to begin the day of my dying"), the right decision and the good decision would be in conflict. What we have, then, at the moment of clinical truth, is an intersection of value systems which is the central and focal problem of medical ethics.

The Caring Ethic

Today, the moment of clinical truth at the intersection of value systems must be faced without the traditional security of a noble, unfailing, universally honored code of ethics. The recent revision of the AMA Code, as well as the Hippocratic Oath and the many codes derived from it, are useful, but they are inadequate for the most crucial ethical question of our day: How do we assure that moral choices, among and between persons whose values and ethical systems may vary widely, can be made in a morally defensible way? How do we preserve our personal moral accountability in a pluralistic society, and assure our patients that we will respect them as moral agents.

Without deprecating various codes, we must recognize that they have lost some of their force because they presuppose a homogeneity of philosophical and theological values that is no longer the case. With so many differences at so many fundamental levels, is medical ethics doomed to atomization? I do not believe so. Despite the greater complexity of clinical decisions in a democratic and pluralistic society, the realities of being ill and being healed (or cared for) have not and will not change fundamentally.

To care for a patient in the full and integral sense I have outlined requires a reconstruction of medical ethics, one that attends to the concept of care in its broadest sense and, indeed, makes caring a moral obligation. There are three requirements for a reconstruction of medical ethics that, I believe, are capable of confronting some of the dilemmas of today's clinical decisions and professional ethics. They define the conditions for an effective reconstruction of the edifice of medical ethics:

1. Such an ethic must be approached in a modular fashion.

2. It must incorporate a clear notion of the "good" of the patient.

3. It must refurbish the concept of profession.

Edmund D. Pellegrino

MODULAR APPROACH TO MEDICAL MORALS

We have long been accustomed to thinking of medical ethics in terms of a uniform code or as a single set of self-contained, self-justifying principles. The erosion of a common philosophical and theological belief system makes this concept no longer tenable. Instead, a complete medical ethics consists of four modular components, closely linked and interdependent, to be sure, yet separable in actual ethical discourse and moral choice.

The first module consists of the positions we take on specific ethical issues of the day: euthanasia, abortion, terminating treatment, living wills, artificial insemination—any of the multitude of new questions that technological capability puts before us. Much of the strife of ethical discourse and decision arises from opposing positions on these issues. Most people simply assert their positions as "right" and "good," and reject argumentation that exposes the sources of their opinions.

The second module contains the philosophical sources upon which the positions in the first module are based. These are in three large categories: (1) the theory of ethics to which we subscribe: deontological, utilitarian, contractarian, consequentialist, or teleological; (2) the construal we place on the fundamental ethical principles of truth-telling, promise-keeping, beneficence, nonmaleficence, justice, and the like; and (3) our concept of the nature, destiny, and worth of human existence.

The third module comprises our theological and religious beliefs: what we think about God, our duties to Him, and the ultimate destiny and meaning of human existence. Believers and nonbelievers alike take positive or negative positions on these questions which seriously affect their moral choices.

The fourth module is less well developed than the other three. Unlike them, it is not substantive in content, but deals with the ethics of the process of interpersonal moral decision making. It comprises our positions on such things as patient participation, strong and weak paternalism, libertarianism, protecting the autonomy and moral agency of the patient, telling the truth, manipulating consent, and handling conflicts between the interacting parties (physicians, other members of the health professions, patients, and their families). This module should aim at assuring a morally defensible transaction between persons who may differ widely on the substantive ethical issues, yet must enter a medical transaction with each other. This is the ethics of a moral relationship between physicians and patients, irrespective of their positions on specific medical-moral questions.

Out of the interaction between these four modules of medical ethics we arrive at what we think is right and good in a particular clinical situation. A complete and mature medical morality requires us to be clear about our positions in each module. Only then can we understand the basis for our actions, and where and at what level we disagree or agree with patients (and others) in clinical decisions.

It is unlikely that we will ever again enjoy wide agreement on the philosophical or theological sources of our medical morality. It is therefore unlikely that we can achieve general agreement on specific clinical-moral decisions. If any common principles are possible, they will probably be deducible only in the fourth component, in a procedural ethics which respects the obligations of each person to be faithful to his or her belief systems.

Development of this fourth module is our most urgent need in medical ethics in a democratic society. The Hippocratic corpus says very little about the process of making decisions. If anything, it is strongly paternalistic, and even warns against sharing information with the patient. The most recent revision of the AMA Code is silent on this subject, though it is treated under the heading of consent in "Opinions of the Judicial Council."[5] On the whole, the most vexing questions about who decides, and how, are still left largely to individual interpretation. This deficiency is no longer acceptable. Patients and their families want to know how we will make our decisions, who will have the final say, and how we will handle potential conflicts. Also, they will increasingly want to know our position on the major medical-moral questions. This is becoming a major issue on the agenda of medical ethics.

"GOOD OF THE PATIENT" CONCEPT

Any ethics of the process of clinical decision must begin with a clear notion of the good of the patient. This is a complex notion, to which it is easy to give superficial assent. All too often, it is little more than a rhetorical device. It is rarely carefully analyzed, yet it is the final criterion of whether a decision is morally sound. It is therefore the unifying theme of all medical ethics, and particularly of any ethics of moral choice and decision making.[6]

The good of the patient is a compound notion, with at least three components which can sometimes be in conflict with each other. A morally good clinical decision should attend to all three senses of patient good and satisfactorily resolve conflicts among them.

Biomedical Good. This is the good a medical intervention can offer by modifying the natural history of disease in a patient. It can be cure, prevention or containment of disease, amelioration of symptoms, or prolongation of life. It is the good aimed at by the doctor's craftsmanship and the result of scientifically correct decisions about what can be done and carrying it out safely, competently, and with minimal discomfort. An intervention that can effectively alter the natural history of the disease is "medically indicated." For the purpose of this discussion, *biomedical good* is synonymous with *medical indication*.

Characteristically, physicians make two errors with respect to medical indications. The first is to reduce the whole of patient good to medical indication. This leads to the fallacy of the medical imperative: if any good can be achieved by a procedure, that procedure must be done. On this view, medical ethics is reduced to doing whatever is medically indicated; and any other sense of the good of the patient is ignored.

The second error is to mix quality-of-life assessments with medical indications. On this view, a treatment or procedure is judged not only by what it can do to change the natural history of a disease, but by the kind of life that results in a particular patient. On this view, some external observer's opinion—the physician's—of the worthwhileness of another person's life is used to deny treatment. This is an unjustifiable mingling of categories of judgment. Whether someone's life is worth living is not measurable by medical means, and therefore it is not the doctor's prerogative to determine. The physician should define, as accurately and objectively as possible, what kind of life might result from treatment, so that the patient (or surrogate) can determine whether it is worth living. This determination should not, of course, be colored by nonmedical value judgments in arriving at medical indication.

Patient's Concept of His/Her Own Good. A biomedically good decision is scientifically correct, but is not automatically a good decision from the patient's point of view. It must be placed within the context of the patient's life situation and value system. It must square with what the patient thinks is "worthwhile," given the circumstances and choices forced by illness. Only the patient can weigh the probable medical benefits of treatment against pain, disability, and loss of dignity that those benefits may "cost" him, or against some ultimate good such as his concept of his own spiritual destiny. Only the patient (or proxy) can determine whether the quality of life predicted by the physician is worthwhile. The range of satisfactions of the sick and disabled is narrowed, but what is left may still be savored by the patient.

When the patient is competent, he can himself ascertain what is in his "best interests." When he is not, his surrogates must ascertain, as closely as possible, what the patient would have taken to be his best interests, were he able to make the choice himself.

The patient's interest, defined in this way, is necessarily subjective and relative. It is the patient's best estimate of what he thinks is good for him, and we cannot know what it is until we ask the patient. This does not deny the fact that some objects of patient interest might be inferred incorrectly, or might conflict with biomedical good or with what others may deem to be in the patient's interest.

The Good of the Patient as a Person. The third sense of "patient good" is the good most proper to being a human. Philosophers argue endlessly about what constitutes the distinguishing feature of being human: freedom, rationality, consciousness, capacity for language, art, or culture. Without trying to settle these debates, it would be hard to deny that one observable feature unique to humans is the capacity to make choices, to set up a life plan, and to determine one's goals for a satisfactory life (among the many possible ways to conduct a human life).

The Caring Ethic

The good that is proper to humans *as* humans is that which fulfills our potentialities as individuals of a rational nature, capable of choice. To be treated as humans is to be accorded the dignity of choosing what we believe to be good and to be accountable for our wrong choices. We cannot exercise our humanity fully unless we are free to make our own mistakes.

The good that is peculiar to being human is the freedom to express our humanity in a choice which is our own. That choice may be right or wrong: what a reasonable person might or might not do. It might, or might not, square with the doctor's concept of good. That it is the patient's good does not make it good in an absolute sense, but we violate a greater good if we do not allow a person to choose.

SOCIAL GOOD

As the cumulative effects of individual medical decision alter the world's demography and high technology consumes an ever larger percentage of our resources, the good of society comes more and more into conflict with the good of the patient. The economic and social costs of prolonging lives of infants, as well as the aged and disabled, are intruding themselves into clinical decisions. A growing body of critics takes physicians to task for exalting individual patient good over that of society. Yet that is the commitment the patient expects.

Are we justified in violating that trust, without changing the explicit promise we make to help the patient? Can physicians be agents of social and fiscal good, and still serve the three senses of patient good which I have described? In the years immediately ahead, this will be perhaps the most vexing dilemma the physician will face.

23

ETHICS OF THE PROCESS OF CLINICAL MORAL CHOICE

The possibilities of conflict between these various components of "the good of the patient" underscore the need for a careful definition of *which* good we mean in defending a specific clinical decision. It also implies some ranking of these various senses of patient good. This is a subject of its own, and I can only suggest an order.

The highest sense of the good of competent patients is that which preserves their capacity to act in a fully human way—that is, to express and act on their perception of their own good. That good is owed all patients, simply because they are human. If a patient is not competent, a surrogate or proxy is expected to ascertain what choice the patient *would* have made. A patient's freedom to choose is limited only when it poses a direct, immediate, and discernible harm to another person, or if fulfilling the patient's perception of good would violate the physician's conscience. The physician is a moral agent, as well as the patient, and cannot be expected to cooperate in what the physician considers to be wrong.

Patients' conceptions of their own good, which rank right behind their good as a human person, take precedence over biomedical good or medical indications. To force medical good on a patient, or to accomplish it by deception or manipulation for the "patient's good," is to violate a patient's good as human being, and as an agent entitled to make moral choices.

Biomedical good and medical indications are therefore lowest in the hierarchy of senses in which we can interpret the good of the patient. Beneficial as they might be, they do not justify violation of the higher good of the patient as a human being to express his or her choices and to determine the specific nature of what is in their "best interests."

The Caring Ethic

An ethics of the process of clinical moral choices, therefore, obligates the physician to respect the several dimensions of the good of the patient and to keep them
distinct and in proper order when they are in conflict.
Some of these obligations are as follows.

In all decisions, the physician has the responsibility for
an objective assessment of biomedical good—that is,
how the proposed treatment will change the short- and
long-term prognosis and history of the disease. That assessment must be objective, scientifically sound, and
free of "quality of life" criteria. In this way, patients or
their surrogates are enabled to determine accurately
what is in the patients' best interests.

Assessment of the good to be achieved by a medical
intervention should be presented to the patient (or surrogate) as sensitively and clearly as possible. It must be
fitted to the patient's educational, cultural, linguistic, and
ethnic background. The physician has an obligation to
assist the patient make as cogent a choice as possible—
and without coercion or deception.

After they have been properly, and sensitively, informed, patients may ask the physician to make the decision for them; and the physician then has a mandate to
do so. Such a mandate is very different from automatically assuming that "the doctor knows what's best" for
the patient and from taking a strangely paternalistic role
from the outset.

With an incompetent (or never-competent) patient,
the physician should accord the same freedom of choice
to surrogates. He has the additional, difficult obligation
to be sure that a surrogate is competent to make the
decision and that the surrogate is acting in the best interests of the patient.

The process is greatly complicated in the case of infants, where the family's wishes and its quality-of-life

determinants may color a decision. But the physician's concern must be the infant, for the infant is the patient, *not* the family. With the never-competent patient, there is no way to ascertain what the patient would see as his or her interests. Therefore medical good—the probability of improving the patient's functioning or comfort—assumes a more dominant place than with the competent or once-competent patient.

When serious moral disagreements between physicians or surrogates occur, and especially in the case of infants, recourse should be had to a judicious, uninvolved, deliberative group—a consultant, an ethics committee, a court-appointed guardian. If all this fails, court intervention may be necessary—but this is not the way to determine what is morally right. It is an inferior way of determining which decision is to be made and to be sure that *some* decision is made that protects legal rights.

The best clinical decisions are those in which medical good, the patient's interests and the freedom to choose are congruent; and in many cases they are. Most often, differences can be "negotiated" if they are approached in trust, without deception and with sensitivity. The quality of the relationship between patients, families, and medical attendants will often be the deciding factor, rather than rules of procedure or moral algorithms.

Unfortunately, the "trust relationship" required for so momentous a decision as, let us say, a no-code order is becoming ever more difficult in contemporary medical care. Team care, multiple consultations, rotations of house staff, institutionalization, stress at the moment of decision—all complicate the relationship. In public and teaching hospitals there is often no one with a sustained relationship with the patient who can serve as a personal physician in the delicate process of making moral choices. This is an intolerable impediment to ethical patient care in the complicated nexus of today's clinical decisions and the reconstruction that medical ethics will demand.

An ethics of moral decision making must include respect for the moral agencies and the moral accountability of all health professionals who interact in the clinical decision. The physician may have technical, and even legal, authority to perform certain acts; the nurse and social worker, authority to perform others; but no one has moral authority over another. Thus all members of medical and health care teams are morally accountable to themselves and to their patients. Each promises to help and to act in the patient's best interests.

There will be times when orders cannot be followed, because the moral principles of some team members are violated. At other times, if a serious transgression of our obligations to patients occurs, "whistle blowing," with all its painful consequences, may be necessary. Physicians need far more awareness of and sensitivity to potentialities for moral conflicts with other health professions, and they must learn to deal with such conflicts in a way which respects the moral agencies of their colleagues.

REFURBISHING THE IDEAL OF A PROFESSION

Our act of profession is the promise we make every time we offer to help a sick person. It declares implicitly, to the patient and family, that we are competent, that we will use our competency in the interests of the patient, and that we can be trusted not to abuse the privileges our promise entails in helping to manage some of the most significant events in a person's life. It allows us, in the patients' interests, to learn all their weaknesses and foibles, to probe, palpate, prick, and incise their bodies—a degree of intimacy that one does not accord strangers.

Edmund D. Pellegrino

No idea has been more debased than the idea of a profession. Today, anyone who undertakes an activity full time, for pay, or with high skill—anyone with special competency or knowledge, anyone with a college degree or credential, anyone who performs some needed service—can call himself a "professional." The list ranges from athletics to astrophysics, from carpentry to salesmanship, from medicine to mortuary science, from pipefitting to politics. Whoever is not an amateur, dilettante, hobbyist, or apprentice is accorded the title "professional."

I have no quarrel with recognition of anyone who pursues excellence in performance, particularly in this age of slovenly craftsmanship. Nor do I wish to preserve the term "professional" for some elite purpose. True elitism is not born of titles anyway, but of the voluntary self-imposition of higher-than-ordinary standards.

Nonetheless, we must not forget that our act of profession as healers is a declaration of commitment—an act of consecration (to use Cushing's word) to a way of life that is not ordinary. It is a promise that we will not place our own interests first, that we will not exploit the vulnerability of those we serve, that we will honor the trust that illness forces upon those who are ill.[7] This necessity for a higher standard impelled Plato to use medicine as his paradigm of the ethical employment of knowledge. Medicine was for him a *tekné*—a craft and art, to be sure, but significantly different from all the others.

Later, in the first century A.D., when the word *profession* was first used by Scribonius Largus, it was tied to a special promise to help humanity and to place it above one's own interests.[8] This has always been the doctor's special promise, his common devotion, and the source for his ethical obligations. When medicine lacks this ethical dimension, it becomes not just a business, trade, or technique, but a betrayal of trust that demeans both the physician and the patient, and leads to angry and satirical attacks on physicians in the world's literature. Pomposity, callousness, and cupidity are common human failings, but they elicit special rancor in physicians because our severest critics expect better of us.

The most corrosive force is still abuse by physicians of the trust that the nature of their duties demands. We must *merit* the trust our act of profession invites. If we do not rise to those obligations, we can hardly protest when we are satirized, treated as trades- or businessmen, and regulated as such. Moral credibility is ours to establish and ours to lose. We cannot blame the FTC, Congress, the media, or the moral standards of society.

The nature of the acts we are expected to perform, together with the trust they demand, form the basis of our professional morality. They are binding on health professionals, even if their philosophical and theological principles differ widely. Only we can determine whether our act of profession is a solemn promise, a contract, a commodity transaction, or a business deal. How we "translate" our act of profession tells more about us than all our rhetoric or codes of ethics.

Our moral choices are more difficult, more subtle, and more controversial than those our profession faced previously. We must make them without the heritage of shared values that could unify medical ethics. Our task is not to abandon hope in medical ethics but to undertake what Camus called "the most difficult task of all, to reconsider everything from the ground up, so as to shape a living society inside a dying society."[9]

That task is not demolition of the edifice of medical morality, but its reconstruction along three lines: (1) replacement of a monolithic with a modular structure for medical ethics, with special emphasis on the ethics of making moral choices in clinical decisions; (2) clarification of what we mean when we speak of the "good" of the patient, and setting priority among the several senses in which that term may be taken; and (3) refurbishing the traditional ideal of a profession as truly a "consecration" of our expertise.[10]

The reconstruction I have suggested calls upon all of us in the health professions to attend to the full spectrum of meanings of the word *care*. Care is the moral base upon which our professional obligations, our ethics, are to be re-formed. Caring, instead of a narrow concept, becomes synonymous with what we are all about, each in our own way. It is also the "common devotion" of all health professionals—the overriding consideration that should bind us in an enterprise that transcends the self-interests of our individual professions.

Sally A.   **2. Nurse and Patient:**

Gadow   **The Caring**

                Relationship

        The spectacular rise of technology in health care has cast a shadow on the image of caring, especially caring that is posited as the essence of a professional relationship. Caring now has connotations like that of hospice, that is, taking care that patients are not abandoned when hope of cure is abandoned. While hope remains, however, it is not caring that will achieve a cure; it is technical expertise that repairs the valve or adjusts the dialysis. Caring, while making patients feel more comfortable, perhaps even cherished, will not arrest pathology; thus it is not allowed to divert time and energy that can be invested in cure. Where there is no conflict between the two, it is because cure is impossible. When conflict arises, cure has priority.

        In the discussion that follows I address two issues that arise for the nurse-patient relationship in light of the care-cure distinction. I then propose two examples of nursing approaches that offer resolution of those issues in a caring relationship.

31

CARING AS A MORAL IDEAL

The first issue involves the nature of caring. What does it mean to describe the nurse-patient dyad as "a caring relationship"? Is caring a moral ideal, rather than a set of behaviors; and if an ideal, does it commit the nurse to certain approaches while prohibiting others?

The image of the caring person is of one who is solicitous, tender, sympathetic, supportive.[1] To describe the nurse-patient relationship as essentially one of caring might then require those traits of nurses rather than others like detachment or efficiency.

I suggest that this is a trivial notion of both caring and nursing, if we are endeavoring to establish the moral essence of the nurse-patient relationship. Certainly the traits are useful; they are part of a technology of interaction that has been refined to an awesome extent but that is only a means, not an end (unless we are willing to reduce nursing to technique for its own sake). Caring as a moral ideal, rather than as an interpersonal technique, entails a commitment to a particular end. That end, I am proposing, is the protection and enhancement of human dignity. Caring as the moral ideal of nursing is concern, above all, for the dignity of patients.

Dignity, too, has its trivial definitions—not because they are inane but because they are fragments portrayed as the whole. Closing the curtains around a patient's bed during an examination, allowing patients to wear their own clothes, allowing them finally to die, by removing the machines, illustrate a current ideology of privacy more than a substantive concept of dignity.

What does a richer meaning of dignity involve? Simply expressed, a being has dignity when it gives to itself its meaning and so creates for itself integrity. Integrity thus implies both the coherence which meaning gives to experience and the origin of that meaning within, rather than outside, the individual.

Dignity here must be understood in the broadest sense—wider, certainly, than the narrow, technical meanings of "ego integrity" from developmental psychology. Reduced to those meanings, few sick persons retain their dignity, and we could make no sense at all of the integrity of infants and comatose persons.

It is perhaps easiest to recognize integrity when it is expressed in the language of verbal assertion ("I want no heroics"; "I want to live until my grandchild is born"; "I'll take my chances living alone because I don't want to depend on anybody"). But in patients who are silent in this regard, dignity must be recognized and affirmed in other forms. One form—described by Robert Burt in relation to patients like Joseph Saikewicz, with an IQ of 10, and Karen Quinlan, in seemingly permanent unconsciousness—is the power of even nonexpressive patients to call forth from their caregivers a response as intense as any verbal patient could evoke. In a chapter titled "Conversation with Silent Patients," he argues that in genuine and therefore agonizing discussion about such patients, each participant in the discussion inevitably would recognize

the futility of attempting to pretend that anyone was powerless . . . even including the apparently silent partner, the comatose or retarded person whose true psychological power over each of the others would be given voice by the cacophony of voices consulted.[2]

Caring, defined as a commitment to protecting and enhancing the dignity of patients, can be described in another way that further identifies it as a distinct moral position: caring is attending to the "objectness" of persons without reducing them to the moral status of objects. By *objectness* I mean the aspects of a person that have been objectified: lifted out of the lived immediacy of experience—objectified either by the individual's designation of a health condition as personally problematic or by the application of a conceptual paradigm that abstracts the condition from the individual in order to address it as an instance of a disease category.

Both forms of objectification have as their end, if not elimination of the condition, at least alleviation of its problematic character for the individual, that is, alleviation of the indignity the condition creates through its disruption of integrity. Therapeutic efforts toward that end necessarily address the objectness of the person. To do so while at the same time, and above all, protecting the patient from being reduced to an object, is to engage in a caring relationship.

The description of caring as a relationship in which patients are protected from being reduced to the moral status of objects leads to the second issue that must be addressed, and in examining that issue the discussion will elaborate the "objectness" of patients and the caring of nurses more concretely.

TECHNOLOGY AND THE OBJECT PARADIGM

The question that now requires an answer is this: Are there aspects of curing that are contrary to caring? Is caring a moral ideal that conflicts with curing in a fundamental way? To put the question in more current terms, Is technology—the symbol of modern curing—an intrinsic violation of dignity?

The answer from the naturalist quarter is yes. The by now almost trite example is the belief that "death with dignity" precludes the use of elaborate technology. Resuscitative and intensive care measures are cited as evidence of the violation that technology has spawned.

The view that machine-supported life is unnatural, a violation of the body's integrity and thus an indignity, can be shown to be mistaken at several levels.[3] However, it points to the phenomenon that is the basis of indignity, allowing us to identify the various ways in which technology is capable of reducing persons to objects.

The violation attributed to technology is a function of the otherness experienced in relation to objects that resist integration into the personal sphere.[4] Objects like animals, computers, and bureaucracies seem to have a life of their own. They are radically other; they resist being assimilated into the integrity of a human life. A complicated network of machinery like an intensive care unit is felt to be more alien to human dignity than non-mechanical forms of care. This is not because the technology is an inherent indignity, and other care is not; it is because apparatus, complicated enough to have a seeming reality of its own, asserts its otherness more emphatically than does a simple apparatus that requires continuous human involvement for its operation.[5]

The reason, then, that technology poses a greater threat to dignity than does less complex care is related to the experience of otherness. Mundane care and simple apparatus involve measures that persons usually can manage for themselves. But complicated measures and machinery are more disruptive; they can remove the locus of control and of meaning from the individual by imposing otherness in two forms, the machine and the professional: (1) the apparatus asserts an otherness that cannot be ignored or easily integrated into the physical or psychological being of the person, and (2) complex techniques require greater expertise than many persons possess, and professionals may be called in to manage the procedure.

Both elements of otherness, the apparatus and the expert, threaten to disrupt personal integrity—and thus to violate dignity—by removing patients from the center of their experience. And precisely to the extent that their dignity is diminished, they are reduced to the status of objects.

In addition to the domination by apparatus and by experts that can accompany the use of technology, patients can be reduced to objects in a more fundamental way than by the use of machines: in the view of the body as a machine. Such reduction occurs because regard for the body exclusively as a scientific object negates the validity of subjective meanings of the person's experience. Those meanings are categorically nonexistent in the scientific object. Thus clinical decisions are based upon external interpretations, not upon the meanings and coherence of the body as constituted by the patient. As scientific object, a body belongs to no particular patient, for such objects have no subjectivity, no self. (The apparatus of mental cogs and gears that is sometimes posited as the self is of course as much a scientific object as the pancreas.)

On this view, in its extreme form (in which the person is reduced to the body and the body to a mechanism), the violation occurs in the negation of the possibility of integrity—a violation more profound than the intrusion of machines and experts. The technology of curing, then, is not the greatest threat to dignity; it is merely a symptom of the violation inherent in the mechanistic paradigm within which technology is employed.[6] In short, the escalating use of apparatus in health care is but an extension of the view of the patient as an apparatus.

Technology is not the cause of our alienation from the world of our experience. It is the friendly symptom without which our malady would be invisible, and thus beyond treatment. Technology merely exhibits our malaise and opens the possibility of cure.[7]

Now that technology displays so vividly the reduction of persons to their objectness, what are the alternatives? I assume that one alternative we would not accept, either as professionals or as patients, is to relinquish the objectifying mode of addressing health problems. The dilemma then becomes enacting a moral commitment to dignity while attending to the objectness of persons. Are concrete approaches entailed by the ideal of caring that might resolve the dilemma? Two approaches suggest themselves as means of affirming the integrity of patients, one having to do with truth, the other with touch.

TRUTH TELLING

The movement toward greater patient autonomy in treatment decisions is one way in which the view of patients as objects has been countered. Disclosure of information to patients is of course central in most cases to their exercise of autonomy. But disclosure can be ambiguous. It can have—as easily as deception—a paternalistic basis, that is, the belief that the truth is good for patients, whether or not they agree. When patients are "treated" with information for its therapeutic value, irrespective of their wishes, they are addressed as objects, as clearly as when other treatment is administered without their consent.

A more subtle belief, generally underlying disclosure practices, also expresses a view of patients as objects. This is the belief that the truth to be disclosed (or withheld) is constituted entirely on the side of the caregiver, consisting of objective information, statistically ordered if possible. Implicit in this view is the belief that the truth of a situation exists independently of the persons involved and, like an experimental drug, is accessible only to the professional, who may offer it to the patient, who in turn can accept or refuse it.

A different view of truth is entailed by commitment to dignity, viz., truth as the most comprehensive and most personally meaningful interpretation of the situation possible, encompassing subjective as well as objective realities, idiosyncratic as well as statistical tendencies, emotional as well as intellectual responses.[8] The opposite of a truth that exists independently of the persons involved, it is a truth that is constituted anew by the patient and professional together, in each situation. Thus it is not accessible originally to the nurse, only then to be disclosed to the patient. Of course, abstract probabilities and clinical findings are disclosed, but whether these define the situation for the patient—whether they are to constitute the truth of the situation in the patient's terms—is not known either to the nurse or the patient until the patient has been assisted to make that determination. The unveiling of a pre-existing truth, the formulation of which involves nothing of the patient's subjectivity, is a form of truth telling consistent with a view of the patient as object. In contrast, assistance to patients in defining their situation and in constituting their personal truth is the approach of caring, an affirmation of the subjectivity of persons that distinguishes them from objects.

This concept of truth is more complex than the simplistic issue "to tell or not to tell" suggests. Because the truth cannot be presented in a "finished" form to patients, but requires their participation in constituting it, the subjectivity not only of the patient but also of the nurse must be engaged. The ideal of caring is an ideal of intersubjectivity, in which both nurse and patient are involved. This means that the values and views of the nurse, though not decisive, are potentially as relevant as those of the patient.

Withholding the nurse's personal view from a patient who inquires is another form of censoring information, according to its therapeutic value, and thereby negating the primacy of patients' involvement in forming their own understanding of the situation. Refusing to allow the nurse's subjectivity to be engaged by a patient is, in effect, refusal to recognize the validity of the patient's subjectivity. The alternative to caring as intersubjectivity is not simply reduction of the patient to an object, but reduction of the nurse to that level as well. Disclosure of the nurse's values not only provides patients another view they may wish to consider, it expresses the nurse's commitment to integrity as the creation of meaning. To the extent that the patient is to be assisted in that process, the nurse too must participate, out of personal dignity— a coherent wholeness from which parts of the self are not deliberately excluded.[9]

SUBJECTIVITY AND TOUCH

The paradox in illness is that concern for the patient as a being with subjectivity, and hence with the dignity that a mere object never can have, often occurs together with impairment severe enough to require assistance with the most intimate activities: breathing, eating, excreting. Yet dignity and dependence need not conflict. Dependence upon another for care of the body constitutes an indignity only when the person cared for becomes an object for the caregiver. In reality, physical care from another presents a possibility for dignity greater than if a patient were capable of independent self-care. Ministrations of care are crucial of course to the physical comfort and, thus, the integrity of the individual by preventing the body's distress from overwhelming the person. But in addition, physical care is important in symbolic ways, and that importance is founded upon the phenomenon of touch.[10]

Among all forms of human interaction, touch is the reminder that objectivity is not even skin deep. In touch, subjectivity exists at the *surface* of the body, and health professionals understand this perfectly. The calling forth of the self in touch is so immediate and potent that elaborate distancing mechanisms are maintained in touch situations in which persons need or wish to remain psychically separate. Both patient and professional tend to regard the patient's body as an object (and the professional's body as an instrument) in order that no bond be created or subjectivity invoked by touching. Technology provides a significant barrier in this respect. The stethoscope is safer than the ear to the chest, and the monitor, with remote viewer, removes the dangers of touching altogether.

Touch is a more compelling form of contact than sight or hearing, because it is the symbol of vulnerability.[11] Touch exposes, in the words of the poet, "the soul unshelled"; it is the dissolution of boundaries.[12] When touch occurs without the devices that neutralize its potency, it offers the supreme risk in an individualistic society: that one person's subjectivity will flow into another's. It is this possibility, however, that makes it a means of overcoming the objectness to which persons (professionals as well as patients) can be reduced in health care.

In the caring relationship, the body is regarded—and touched—by the nurse as the immediate, lived reality of the patient. This entails a breach of objectivity: empathic touch affirms, rather than ignores, the subjective significance of the body for the patient. Its purpose is not palpation or manipulation but expression—an expression of the nurse's participation in the patient's experience. Because subjective involvement in another's suffering is possible only where concern exists, empathic touch is concern made tangible.

The caring relationship not only overcomes *objectivity* by touching the self of the patient, it alleviates the isolation of pure *subjectivity*. Since it is, after all, impossible for persons to regard themselves strictly as objects, one defense of patients against the objective paradigm is the other extreme, equally alienating in the opposite direction: retreat into self. The poet Auden describes men in a surgical ward:

They are and suffer; that is all they do;
A bandage hides the place where each is living,
His knowledge of the world restricted to
The treatment that the instruments are giving.[13]

The intersubjectivity that touch restores is an alternative to both extremes. It reaches past the objectivity of treatment ("the treatment that the instruments are giving"), allowing the patient, in turn, to reach out of the solitude of suffering ("the place where each is living").

The meanings of touch are not limited to empathic expression. Touch can be used instrumentally—literally as a substitute for instruments—to locate and correct pathology. This is its use in a wide spectrum of health measures, from the delicate fingering of an aneurysm to the mystical transmission of healing forces. There is, in short, a technology of touch, in which nothing is expressed from one person to another. Patients are not necessarily reduced to objects, but neither is their subjectivity engaged.

41

Still another form of touch is neither empathic nor instrumental; it is intrinsically demeaning precisely because, paradoxically, its intent is to bestow dignity. This use of touch can be described as "philanthropic" because of the asymmetry it assumes: "sufficiency and independence on one side and needy dependence on the other."[14] In philanthropy, touch is a gift from one who is whole to one who is not. The real indignity here is not the "needy dependence" in the other but its denial in oneself, in the giver. It is the "helping of the brother who can in no way be oneself" that demeans, first by equating need with indignity and then by removing oneself from both.[15] In the philanthropic model, touch marks the person as untouchable, proposing at the same time to redress the indignity it creates.

In the caring relationship, the subjectivity of the patient is assumed to be as whole and valid as that of the nurse. Their intersubjectivity, described by Buber as dialogue, is a relation

—no matter whether spoken or silent—where each of the participants really has in mind the other or others in their present and particular being and turns to them with the intention of establishing a living mutual relation.[16]

The typical objection to a relation of dialogue in health care is that it asks too much of the patient, who cannot be expected to give to the caregiver. In reply, it has to be pointed out that this is the same asymmetry that philanthropy assumes. In fact, however, even on that model, patients are expected to offer the professional a gift—a gift of inestimable value, without which even the most one-sided relationship collapses: the gift of trust. Both sides, as it turns out, have something of value to give the other—a fact overlooked also in the mechanistic paradigm. There, too, the body first has to be entrusted to the professional in order for cure to proceed, and the professional, even while reducing the person to an object, redeems that reduction by attempting to restore a level of function that is consonant with the patient's subjective values.

The means as well as the ends of health care—in either a mechanistic or a philanthropic paradigm—already presuppose a significant degree of intersubjectivity. In those models, however, it remains secondary. In the empathic or caring ideal, that mutuality becomes the moral foundation of nursing: commitment to the dignity that distinguishes persons from objects. In the modern clinical context, in which objectness so easily undermines dignity, empathic touch becomes a means of continually reestablishing the mutuality in which patients then are affirmed as persons, rather than objects. And as *persons*, patients are free to determine the formulations of truth that are compatible with their individual meanings of dignity.

Mila Ann
Aroskar

3. Ethical Relationships between Nurses and Physicians: Goals and Realities—A Nursing Perspective

*A brief conversation with a physi-*cian colleague about relationships between physicians and nurses led him to conclude that nurse-physician relationships boil down to "how they interact with each other." While we might all agree on this observation, it does not take us very far in sorting out and understanding the broad spectrum of more or less ethical relationships between physicians and nurses. They range from nonexistent, through master-servant, the adversarial, to collegial.

The National Commission on Nursing reported in 1981 that a major category of issues in nursing is "relationships among nursing, medical staff, and hospital administration, including nurses' ability to participate through organizational structures in decision-making as it relates to nursing care, the value and development of collegial relationships among health care professionals."[1] Characterized as a fundamental unresolved issue is lack of recognition for nurses' worth in patient care.

Assumptions of this paper include, but are not necessarily limited to, the following:

Ethical Relationships

1. Ethical relationships between nurses and physicians are a good, to be sought insofar as they enhance nurse-patient-physician interactions (and respect for persons).
2. Areas of conflict in male-female relationships such as power and authority are at stake in nurse-physician interactions in both covert and overt ways.
3. Health care professionals are interdependent.
4. There are significant obstacles, such as historic, social, psychologic, economic, and philosophic, to the achievement of ethical relationships between nurses and physicians in health care systems.
5. Practicing nurses and physicians are competent adults who are responsible for personal and professional choices and actions.

Ethical relationships and interactions between nurses and physicians are characterized for this paper in the following four ways:

1. Mutual respect, based on the inherent worth of all participants in nurse/physician relationships.
2. Individuals in nurse/physician relationships are never used only as means to ends decided upon solely by others.
3. Explicit recognition that each participant has significant contributions to make in enhancement of quality patient care.
4. Major decisions, related directly and indirectly to patient care, are made with explicit input from all who carry out the decisions and are affected by the decisions.

These criteria for ethical relationships and interactions between nurses and physicians lead to the observation that many nurse-physician relationships or interactions are not ethical. This is a troubling conclusion for individuals who are involved personally—for decision-making processes, for the medical and nursing professions, and for the organizational structures within which medical and health care are delivered.

OBSTACLES TO ETHICAL RELATIONSHIPS

I turn now to a more specific (though brief) consideration of the obstacles to ethical relationships and interactions between nurses and physicians. Knowledge of these obstacles may contribute to a sense of despair or to more explicit recognition of the dimensions of the challenge that face anyone who seeks a "quick fix" to the unethical relationships that negate respect for health care professionals and their contributions to patient care.

Experience of the Work World. Nurse-physician relationships are complicated by the multiplicity of individuals with whom each must interact in complex health care settings. For example, nurses work with house staff, private physicians, medical students, and consulting physicians. Physicians work with multiple levels of nursing staff, such as aides, assistants, practical nurses, registered nurses (with an RN and several varieties of education preparation), clinical nurse specialists, and a nursing administrative hierarchy. In addition, nurses and physicians—according to a nurse-medical sociologist, Timothy Sheard—work in contrasting worlds of underlying logic and lived experience. Ignoring these differences is to assume, incorrectly, that nurses and physicians inhabit identical work worlds.

Ethical Relationships

Individual nurses and physicians may experience any or all of the differences in varying degrees, depending on their settings and sensitivities to multiple realities. They explain, to some degree, the often expressed frustrations of both nurses and physicians, as they seek goals of patient welfare, from differing experiences and views of the work world. These can lead to disagreement about patient-care decisions and to adversarial standoffs that contribute to stress and further conflict.

The six work dimensions on which nurses and physicians differ are sense of time, sense of resources, unit of analysis, work assignment, rewards, and sense of mastery.[2]

Sheard claims that physicians have an enduring sense of time which constricts and expands to match patient problems. Time is considered not in hours but by the course of illness, as the patient progresses toward recovery, stabilization of chronic illness, or death. This is contrasted with nurses' sense of hourly, strictly scheduled time, with work organized around scheduling of tasks. Interruptions in work routines, such as those incurred when physicians order medications to be given at odd times, are resented as disruptions. Nurses may have to give such medications late, or at routine times, in order to facilitate the work flow. Physicians rarely appreciate what a *stat* (immediate) order may mean to one on a routine schedule, since physicians don't think in terms of a rigid work schedule. In short, there is little understanding of the rationale underlying either's organization of work time.

Nurses have a "scarcity view" of hospital resources, as limited and difficult to obtain. Frequently, they meet resistance from supply and information departments, and have too much work to complete in an eight-hour day; so they try to eliminate tasks which appear unnecessary.

The nurse is caught in the middle as he or she struggles to provide the bridge between written and executed orders—while the physician, with an "abundance view" of hospital resources, writes orders in the patients' charts with little sense of the time and difficulty involved in carrying them out. There are several reasons for this, such as the hospital's applying few sanctions against physicians who request unnecessary tests or treatments; physicians' writing requests easily, with little or no involvement in obtaining supplies or test results; or physicians' desire to master new tests and techniques.

Physicians use a "global" unit of analysis, organizing all data around the individual patient, while nurses use a particulate unit of analysis, with more emphasis on completion of scheduled tasks than on the patient's overall health problems and progress. Nurses often lack an integrated sense of the relationship between a particular task and the patient's well-being. Work assignments differ in that physicians deal with patients by case, whereas nurses are assigned geographically, with less continuity of patient care in many settings (primary nursing to the contrary). This type of nursing assignment, as well as shorter hospital stays, prevents nurses (who are so assigned) from developing an ongoing therapeutic relationship with patients.

Physicians and nurses also differ in terms of rewards within the system. While physicians are paid a salary or fee for service, nurses are paid an hourly wage, like most laborers. This means of reimbursement reinforces the sense that nurses' work consists of a specified number of hours of work and erodes dedication to service and a sense of professionalism among nurses, who experience this as part of their work world.

Physicians, according to Sheard, have a strong sense of mastery over their work, derived from the integrated structure of their work, such as responsibility for cases and tasks organized around individual patients, which adds to a sense of relationship between tasks and the patient's condition.[3] Nurses have a weaker sense of mastery over their work, stemming from difficulties in administering the machinery of hospital bureaucracy, their particulate view of tasks (rather than patients), and their shifting assignments, which prevents the development of patient relationships. The functional division of labor in nursing and the hourly wage combine to weaken a nurse's sense of mastery over work. This contributes to a sense of powerlessness in the system.

Lack of understanding the ways in which physicians and nurses experience their work worlds probably contributes more to frustration and misunderstandings in physician-nurse relationships than many realize. These are aspects of the context which contribute to the difficulty in developing more ethical relationships.

An insight from Gilligan's research in moral development bears consideration as we reflect on obstacles to achieving more ethical relationships between and among physicians and nurses, individually and collectively. This research has been developed out of Kohlberg's work on levels of moral development. Individual moral development influences how men and women, nurses and physicians, think about and make decisions and interact. Also, it affects whether one thinks reflection on relationships among nurses and physicians is a worthwhile effort!

Gilligan's research found that women construct moral problems differently from the way men perceive and construct them. Moral problems, for women, arise from conflicting responsibilities rather than competing rights. Resolution of moral problems requires a mode of thinking that is more contextual and narrative, with an overriding desire to avoid hurting others rather than a more formal and abstract mode of thinking. This concept of morality, as concerned with the activity of care, centers moral development around the understanding of responsibility and relationships, just as the conception of morality as fairness ties moral development to the understanding of rights and rules.[4]

This is not to say that one conception is better than the other, but suggests that there are differences for men and women in how ethical relationships are viewed and decisions made. They should, at least, be recognized as enhancing or negating the potential for more ethical relationships between nurses and physicians. Such recognition also points out the folly of thinking there is any "quick fix" for bringing about changes in decision-making structures in health care or developing more collegial relationships among nurses and physicians.

Health Care Views. Additional dimensions to the complexity of nurse-physician relationships include views about health care that influence interactions. They also may be considered as models which negate or enhance more ethical relationships between physicians and nurses. Not only do nurses and physicians experience their lived work worlds in dissimilar modes, they may hold different views of health care that increase conflict in interactions and decrease possibilities for development of more ethical relationships.

These views also affect how decision-making processes are perceived, such as control of the processes, who decision makers should be, and who has input into major decisions affecting patient care. These views may also be held by patients, families, administrators, and policy makers, either implicitly or explicitly. The four views, or models, have been adapted from an article by Lisa Newton, a philosopher,[5] as follows:

Ethical Relationships

1. Health care as medical cases or scientific projects, with cure of diseases as the most important goal
2. Health care as honoring patients' rights to services for relief of pain and suffering
3. Health care as a commodity, with cost containment as a major goal
4. Health care as promotion, maintenance, and restoration of an individual's optimum level of health in a caring community

Each of these views or models significantly impacts on if, and how, nurses and physicians interact with each other in terms of enhancing or negating more ethical relationships, according to the criteria stated earlier in this paper.

The view that health care is primarily medical cases or scientific projects, with cure as the most important goal, is the professional, dominant perspective. On this view, health care institutions are primarily a "doctors' workshop," with doctors, rather that patients, the major clients. The physician is viewed as a scientist who carries on projects, with the hospital as the laboratory. In the background, rather like shadows, are nursing and other activities. They exist to facilitate physicians' activities and projects, which are carried on to meet medical goals. Other health care professionals are primarily accountable to physicians, with nurses carrying out doctors' orders and physicians directly and indirectly influencing the delivery of nursing care and services.

This image of the hospital as the physician's workshop is reinforced historically, through the concept of the family as the institutional model for operation of hospitals in the late nineteenth and early twentieth centuries. (This model is still followed at some medical centers with which the author is familiar.) Nurses were conceived of as caring for the "hospital family." Nurses, like mothers, were responsible for meeting the needs of all members of the hospital family. They were expected to serve the needs of physicians, who were free to come and go. Physicians usually did not reside in the household, as nurses often did (i.e., the nurses' residence). When "the men" were absent, nurses were expected to assume full responsibility for decision making by taking on the traditional male role, with this decision-making role relinquished when physicians were available on patient care units. Nurses were, and still are, constantly supportive of the institution, especially of its male members.[6] The view of nursing's primary responsibility, as a preserver and protector of physician and hospital reputations, appears explicitly as late as 1950, in the *ANA Code of Ethics*.

This is a very paternalistic view of health care institutions—with physicians as primary decision makers—and serves to perpetuate the doctor-nurse "game." That is, nurses are expected to make recommendations about patient care while, at the same time, appearing passive, so that it appears that the recommendations are initiated by the physician. It is a version of the male-female game played in societies like ours to reinforce gender stereotypes.[7] This type of game-playing makes open discussion of patient care options and choices impossible and is disrespectful of nurses' contributions to patient care, in the sense that it is not explicitly recognized and considered in patient care decisions.

This indirect communication can be hazardous for patients. Conversation with a nurse (on a renal dialysis unit at a large metropolitan teaching hospital) assured me that the doctor-nurse game is still played, as new physicians come to her unit and wonder aloud what should be done for particular patients. When the nurse tells a physician her recommendation, the physician writes the orders—

which the nurse has given verbally—and signs his name.

For the most part, this negates a relationship between nurses and physicians that respects a nurse's competence and contributions. It makes the nurse something of a "nonperson" in nurse-physician interactions, on which patient welfare is dependent. It is demeaning to physicians and nurses alike, when patient welfare and interests become part of a covert game. (This game is also reminiscent of the master-servant relationship of physicians and nurses that was the title of a nursing-text chapter not many decades ago.) This relationship is unethical because it denies that nurses and physicians, together, have significant contributions to make in patient care, and neither should use the other mainly as a means to an end decided upon by the other. The master-servant relationship should be challenged and questioned whenever and wherever it is recognized in health care settings.

A *second* view of health care is that health care professionals and institutions exist primarily to honor patients' rights to services for relief of pain and suffering, with health care professionals accountable to patients/clients who decide when their pain and suffering are relieved, when they are satisfied with services rendered, and so on. Needs and wants of patients, as identified by patients, predominate in this view, with health care professionals serving more as expert advisors than as primary decision makers. On this view, needs identified by patients, based on their health goals and values, would be decisive.

Patient interests and goals are dominant and explicitly solicited in decision-making processes at various system levels, ranging from decisions about individual patients to input in institutional policymaking through mechanisms such as community boards. Consumer movements, legislative action on the Patients' Bill of Rights (in some states), and some malpractice suits seemed to point in the direction of more consumer control of health and health-care decision making.

This view is at the other end of the spectrum from the first view and raises significant questions about the potential for health care professionals being used as means to patients' ends. Such a worry receives attention in such documents as *Making Health Care Decisions,* volume 1 of the President's Commission for the Study of Ethical Problems in Medicine and Biomedical and Behavioral Research (October 1982). This report on ethical and legal implications of informed consent in patient-practitioner relationships advocates shared decision making. At the same time, it states that patient choice is not absolute. That is, patients are not entitled to insist that health care practitioners provide them services when it "would violate either the bounds of acceptable practice or a professional's own deeply held moral beliefs or would draw on a limited resource on which the patient has no binding claim."[8]

On the other side, the *ANA Code for Nurses with Interpretive Statements* (1976) could be taken as more supportive of the view of health care as dominated by patients' decision making. An emphasis in the 1976 revision of the Code is that nurses are primarily accountable to patients. This view of accountability places nurses who hold this position into adversarial relationships with physicians or nurses who hold the first view. In reality, this view has not posed a major threat to the first view (of physician ownership of decisions in medical care). However, it does not follow that this view is more ethical, according to criteria for ethical relationships as stated by the author.

The *third* view that nurses and physicians might hold is that medical and health care institutions sell their services as commodities, like others in the marketplace. A major goal, on this view, is cost containment for survival purposes, with competition viewed as a primary means to this goal. Health care is "marketed" by hospitals and other health care agencies, with the patient as a consumer or customer. Physicians may be "outside contractors" or institutional employees, as in HMOs. Nurses and other health care professionals are generally employees.

Health care professionals, on this view, are primarily accountable to the administrative hierarchy of the employing institution and to those who make financial and budget decisions. Institutional interests of survival take precedence over competing interests of traditional medical privileges and over patient expectations and needs. Examples of a marketing orientation are seen in hospitals where "packages" of nursing services are developed from which patients make a selection and in states such as Pennsylvania, where some hospitals are competing to start bigger and better programs of emergency life-saving systems as marketing tools to bring in larger numbers of critically ill patients to fill beds.

Marketing of services and assuring payment for services become major focuses for this institution's energies and policy decisions. Other goals and values, which compete with economic and survival interests of the institution, dominate decision making at administrative levels and filter down to patient care units in the form of regulations for patients' days in the hospital, staff reduction (which may endanger patient welfare), and closing—or never opening—patient care units.

Nurses and physicians may be viewed as means to meeting institutional goals, with little consideration or respect for each health care professional's necessary contributions to patient welfare. This view may support even more authoritarian, arbitrary kinds of decision making when economic survival is perceived as the major issue. This view may also lead to more adversarial relationships between health care professionals, when one considers legislative actions such as those in California for delivering health care to the poor and for reimbursing health care providers. (This legislation requires providers to bid against one another for both Medi-Cal patients and the privately insured. Hospitals are required to bargain for contracts to serve Medi-Cal patients, who have been notified to expect care only when it is necessary to protect life or prevent significant disability.)[9] Patient care decisions, based on need and considerations of individual welfare, will be subsumed under a utilitarian mode of decision making based on the consequences of alternative administrative choices that benefit the hospital in terms of institutional competition and survival. This approach conflicts profoundly with the traditional patient-centered ethic with which health care professionals are imbued in their professional education.

This view of health care, primarily as a commodity, negates the claim of something special about availability and accessibility to health care services as a means for individuals to carry out their life plans. The range of decision-making choices is narrowed both for health care providers and patients, and particularly when patients are poor. One thinks of the consequences to the unemployed, who can no longer afford health insurance for themselves and their families, increasing use of mental health services, and the increasing infant mortality rate in the Detroit area.

The struggle for support for health care institutions and their survival has already had undesirable consequences, directly for patients and indirectly for health care professionals whose services are not available to

Ethical Relationships

those in need. Paul Starr, in his book *The Social Transformation of American Medicine* (1982), indicates that the growth of administrative and corporate medicine in this country weakens the sovereignty of the medical profession. Prospects are for greater disunity, inequality, and conflict throughout the entire health care system.[10]

This third view has received extended attention because the author thinks it may become a dominant perspective on health care decisions at institutional levels, negating the goal of more ethical relationships between physicians and nurses, as health care professionals are viewed (with patients) as means to institutional ends. Nurses will be most directly threatened because institutions will perceive themselves as more dependent on physicians' admitting patients than on maintenance of patient care services, such as nursing, that are not revenue producing.

These three views and models of medical and health care, though briefly described, do not enhance the potential for more ethical relationships between physicians and nurses. They all regard nurses as means to others' ends. They do not explicitly enhance recognition of the contributions and decisions by nurses, as they are intertwined with those of physicians in patient care. Also, there is little or no opportunity for enhancement of mutual respect for all who are affected by and involved in major decisions at the patient-care or administrative levels in models in which either physicians, or patients, or administrators are viewed as *the* decision makers, to the exclusion of each other and always of nurses.

The *fourth* view, of health care as promotion, maintenance, and restoration of the individual's optimum level of health in a caring community, offers greater possibilities for ethical nurse-physician relationships and interactions. Hospitals and other health care institutions are considered settings for face-to-face communities. Patients' goals, values, and well-being are the major focus in making decisions. In addition, the goals, values, and expertise of physicians and nurses are explicitly considered in the decision-making processes that directly and indirectly affect patients and impinge on relationships between physicians and nurses. This view implies respect for the contributions and competence of both physicians and nurses in patient care. Neither nurses nor physicians are used primarily as means to others' ends or goals. Nor are nurses simply means to physicians' ends and goals.

This view is more congruent with organization of nursing care delivery in primary nursing modes and with the joint-practice model that far-thinking nurses and physicians have been struggling to bring to reality for more than a decade, in order to deliver more effective and holistic health care. This mode recognizes the interdependence of nurses and physicians and the complementary contributions that each makes to patient care in a variety of settings. Thus the fourth view of health care enhances, rather than negates, ethical relationships between nurses and physicians.

CONCLUSION

Although this last perspective may seem fragile and idealistic, when looked at against the powerful views of professional dominance and administrative-corporate control of decision making, one should consider what is to be lost if we would give up the effort to develop more ethical—that is, more collegial—relationships among nurses and physicians. I cannot think of any moral grounds to support discontinuing the effort. At stake are foundational values and principles in health care that speak to respect for and the inherent worth of persons as individuals and as individuals in community. That is, all who are involved in making decisions that affect colleagues as well as patients—such as "blowing the whistle" on unsafe practices in patient care—are grounded in moral/ethical considerations.

I do not discuss this perspective as something new or as a panacea, but in hope that it will stir our imaginations with the different possibilities for relationships among physicians and nurses. New relationships, I hope, will alter the ways decisions are made, enhancing the possibility for all of us to become more, rather than less, human in systems that are often criticized as inhumane for both patients and providers. The personal and professional integrity of nurses and physicians is at stake.

Thinking about health care systems and institutions as responsive and responsible caring communities leads away from the team rhetoric so widely used as a model for patient care. Erde, a philosopher, in a thoughtful article on team talk in health care, lays the problems out (in sports lingo) to describe norms, goals, and roles that are not congruent with the variety of ways in which teams can be characterized (the sports model being only one). Social norms of the team differ from moral norms. Whistle blowing on a team member is an example where these norms conflict. Social norms require that team members support each other by (among other possibilities) hiding what goes on within the team. Moral norms, on the other hand, may require blowing the whistle on what is viewed as "tattling" by another team member. Erde suggests that team talk seems to hide the real need for change in the hospital by suppressing feelings of alienation or by manipulating people to feel guilty, while the causes of alienation are allowed to continue. He also discusses respect for the separate interests and contributions of all concerned, rather than maintaining the pretense that equality of status exists.[11]

Four criteria for more or better ethical relationships that apply to appraising nurse-physician relationships were stated at the beginning of this paper. Is there evidence that these criteria have any potential for realization? The primary nursing organizational mode (in which one nurse takes responsibility for a small group of patients during their hospitalization) and the President's Commission Report *(Making Health Care Decisions)* have been mentioned.

The author's research on nurses' feelings and attitudes about ethical decision making in intensive care units in a large teaching/research hospital identifies areas in which nurses can and should contribute when such decisions are considered as discontinuing treatment for an individual when cure is no longer possible. This study also found that while decisions are frequently made solely by physicians, they are as often made with input from patients, families, and others. The development of interdisciplinary institutional ethics committees, serving as educational and consultation resources to individuals struggling with difficult ethical decisions and to policymaking groups, is further support for new social arrangements in health care delivery that have the potential for meeting the criteria for ethical relationships. These criteria are mutual respect, based on the inherent worth of all participants in an interaction; recognition that each participant has significant contributions to make in enhancement of quality patient care; making major decisions with explicit input from all who execute and are affected by the decisions; and not using individuals in an interaction solely as means to ends decided upon by others.

Better ethical relationships among nurses and physicians are not an impossible dream. They require sensitivity to the consequences of recognized differences in the lived worlds of nurses and physicians, and in the various views and conflicting models of health care that contribute to adversarial postures among health care professionals. Nurses and physicians should examine, individually and together, their dominant perspectives on nurse-physician relationships and interactions. Consider current policies and institutional structures in terms of their negation or enhancement of the four criteria that respect and support decision making that takes into account the integrity of physicians *and nurses* as interdependent decision makers and contributors to patient welfare.

In summary, this perspective requires knowledge of the different work worlds of physicians and nurses, relinquishing mindsets that negate better ethical nurse-physician relationships, and the active promotion of new mindsets and decision-making structures that enhance ethical nurse-physician relationships in all patient-care settings.

H. *Tristram*
Engelhardt, Jr.

4. Physicians, Patients, Health Care Institutions— and the People in Between: Nurses

The world rarely accords with the neat distinctions our language presupposes in dealing with it. This is somewhat less true in the case of the social world, for we fashion it to reflect our ideas and purposes. However, our purposes, goals, and conceptions are often complex and intertwined. They develop over time, weaving a complexity that even patient analysis can only in part resolve into distinct elements. This is especially the case with regard to the professions. Nursing, medicine, and the law, for example, do not reflect a conceptually unified set of goals and purposes. Rather, they have developed, as do all professions, in response to a series of shifting perceptions of important human tasks. Thus one is likely to have serious difficulty discovering *the* way in which nurses, physicians, or lawyers aid us in coping with the world, caring for other individuals, or curing or resolving problems. This is in part the case because the service goals that determine professions are a heterogeneous accretion of purposes, as much determined by historical accident as clear conceptual necessity. In addition, learned professions possess not only goals directed to societal or client service, but to the development and maintenance of knowledge and skills. This distance between the altruistic and intellectual goals of learned professions introduced a major complicating factor in the description of professions and their relations with their clients. In addition, professions are modes of gaining a livelihood. As a result, they become natural vehicles for developing and protecting special financial and social perquisites. Much of what one associates with being a nurse, physician, or lawyer is a reflection of often long-established social divisions of power, prestige, and financial advantage. This is probably nowhere more true than in the contrast between the positions of nurses and physicians.

Thus I offer a defense of the proposition that differences between the physician-patient and nurse-patient relationship are predominantly accidental outcomes of social distributions of perquisites and powers. There are, I contend, no essential or conceptually significant differences between the professions of nursing and medicine in their caring for patients. One discovers, at best, differences in accent and emphasis. Central to understanding the triad of physicians, nurses, and patients are the conflicts and tensions engendered by the various restraints on power and authority that stem from the prevailing hierarchies in health care institutions.

A part of the confusion attendant to comparing the roles of physicians and nurses stems from the wide range of activities engaged in by physicians and nurses. Physicians, and thus medicine, embrace the activity not only of surgeons and pediatricians, obstetricians, anesthesiologists, and internists, but the undertakings of physicians in preventive medicine, psychiatry, and psychoanalysis as well. As a result, medicine includes activities of surgery, treatment through pharmacological agents, the fashioning of public policy in preventive medicine, and various complex activities of curing and caring undertaken by psychiatrists. Indeed, if one looks at the activities of physicians now and in the past, one sees them playing various roles as curers, as carers, as individuals involved in the prevention of illness, as well as individuals assuming special quasi-priestly roles.

If one looks at this collage of undertakings, it is difficult to find a single sense of medicine. Indeed, if one explores the notion of the medical model, one discovers the same ambiguities. There is a sense of medical model, as contrasted with religious models, of explaining illness and disease. Here one might think of Hippocrates' argument in *The Sacred Disease*, that epilepsy developed from natural causes and should not be seen as having special divine origins. In this sense, there was a competition throughout the Middle Ages between medical and religious models of explaining illness and disease.[1] This sense of "medical" also encompasses nursing.

Other senses of medical model are employed to identify somatic models of explanation, or patho-anatomical and patho-physiological models of explanation, as opposed to psycho-analytic or behavioral models. Finally, in addition to being invoked in identifying models of explanation, the term "medical model" has been used to indicate a particular genre of physician-patient relationships in which the patient is subservient to, and takes orders from, the physician. However, there are many physician-patient relationships that are not "medical" in this sense.

The same range of nursing models exists as well. Nurses engage in their profession as surgical nurses, psychiatric nurses, nurses in intensive care units, or as school nurses. There is, in addition, a wide range of competence among nurses, ranging from nurse practitioners and registered nurses to licensed practical nurses and various nurse auxiliaries. Nursing, as a consequence, spans individuals who possess various levels of scientific knowledge and technological skills. Not only do highly skilled nurses in medical intensive care units nurse individuals back to health, but so do unskilled individuals under less exacting circumstances. Even this weakest sense of nursing has similarities with the suggestions for care offered by Hippocrates in the *Regimen* books.

In any event, the range of activities undertaken by nurses is so extensive that the "nursing model" (whatever that might mean) suffers from the same ambiguities as the term "medical model." Indeed, given the ambiguity and scope of the latter notion, it would appear to encompass not only what physicians do, but what dentists, nurses, occupational therapists, and physical therapists do. At least there is that compass, insofar as the medical model identifies a particular genre of explanation or a particular variety of healer-client relationships.

These ambiguities, one must recognize, are reflected also in the wide range of ways in which one can be a patient. An individual is a patient somewhat differently if he or she comes for coronary bypass surgery, treatment of gonorrhea, long-term treatment of diabetes, routine immunizations, completion of insurance forms, or psychoanalysis. Caring and coping will vary with these contexts, as will the sought-for contribution of physicians and nurses.

If one tries to identify distinctions between nurses and physicians in their approaches to caring for patients, such distinctions may appear difficult to isolate, given this wide range of understandings of what it is to be a physician, nurse, or patient. These difficulties can be circumvented if one explores how the language of disease, illness, sickness, and health is structured. To begin with, descriptions of circumstances as conditions of illness, sickness, disease, or health are always made under two major clusters of presuppositions. The first is a set of values regarding what should count as the range of expectable or normal human functions, of freedom from pain, and of the character of good human form and grace.[2] Though these clusters of values are likely to differ from culture to culture, given different environmental contexts and cultural expectations, there are not likely to be major or at least essentially distinguishing differences between nurses and physicians. The second major cluster of presuppositions involves what counts as proper explanations of illnesses, diseases, sicknesses, and states of health. However, nursing and medicine share the same common views of medical explanation. There are much larger differences between orthodox physicians and chiropractors than between physicians and nurses.

The differences turn on the capacity of physicians and nurses to fashion social reality. Individuals in authority in a society not only describe reality, explain it, and evaluate it, but have an authority to create social roles. Thus, when a physician finds a patient is totally disabled by multiple sclerosis, he or she not only brings a cluster of findings together in a descriptive taxon which reflects certain human evaluations of function and ability, but also certain at least weak explanatory assumptions. The physician casts that individual, as well, within a sick role. As Talcott Parsons indicates, being placed in a sick role excuses an individual from certain responsibilities and establishes certain prima facie social obligations to seek treatment.[3] In addition, patients, through structured systems of third-party reimbursement, social security, and other welfare enterprises, become entitled to particular payments, given particular sorts of diagnoses. Indeed, diagnoses can entail the loss of the right to move freely, as may occur with mental illness. Physicians can create social reality by fashioning a therapy role of a particular sort with canonical social standing. In this sense, physicians are like judges. When a judge says "You are found guilty," the sentence is not to be understood as simply a descriptive statement. It is performative; it creates social reality.

Because of laws requiring a physician's prescription for access to particular drugs, physicians have a further social role in legitimating certain activities. A physician's prescription makes the difference between licit and illicit possession of drugs. A major difference between physicians and nurses turns on the restriction of such performative and enabling functions to physicians. Any attempt to understand the difference between the physician-patient and nurse-patient relationship in our society must take place against the background of these special social powers and perquisites of physicians. Though there are some differences—for example, in the knowledge and abilities of obstetricians versus midwives, anesthesiologists versus nurse-anesthetists, psychiatrists versus psychiatric nurses—the most startling differences are in social protection of a central set of physician privileges regarding the prescription of drugs, the practice of surgery, and the forwarding of diagnoses. Differences in the character of curing and caring by physicians and nurses reflect these special privileges by which physicians restrain trade.

NURSING AND THE LEFTOVERS FROM MEDICINE

To understand the position of nursing in caring for patients, one must realize that nurses have, in their domain of authority, what medicine has left to them. Nursing developed, for the most part, as a profession auxiliary to medicine and health care institutions. For a long period of time, nurses were not considered to be independent agents, able to diagnose or to treat on their own. They were seen as carrying out the orders of physicians and the general routines of hospitals in the care of patients.[4] As such, they were construed as either servants of hospitals or servants of physicians, but rarely, and only in very limited circumstances, as independent agents. One might think of the now famous phrase by which physicians were construed as the "captain of the ship" in *McConnel v. Williams*.[5] Such arguments about the scope of vicarious liability presumed that nurses acted under the direction of physicians or hospital policy, at least in the great proportion of their activities. Indeed, the recent history of nurses is marked by an attempt by their profession to secure the right to make independent diagnoses and institute independent plans of treatment in ever more expanded areas of health care. This development has been marked by a collateral expansion of the liability of nurses.[6]

The history of nursing in the last decade and a half contrasts with the emergence of physician assistants. Physician assistants, in great proportion, function as a substitute for what nurses in the 1970s and 1980s were reluctant to remain: a special auxiliary profession for physicians.[7] Indeed, the education of physician assistants is often predicated upon selecting individuals who will work well under the direction of physicians and not seek to make independent choices outside the direction of physicians who employ them. It is ironic that, as the nursing practitioner movement begins, physician assistants appear. The interest of nurses to act as an independent profession, perhaps strengthened by the women's liberation movement of the 1970s, caused nursing to pursue a line of development that led to the profession of physician assistants to fill the vacuum.

It would be interesting to compare in detail the ways in which physician assistants are employed as physician "extenders," with a view to affording patients more contact with health care providers, versus the roles of nurses. Surely, in part, physician assistants contribute to the amount of caring and time available to aid patients in coping with their problems. Physician assistants in many ways play roles analogous to those of nurses, at least in a range of settings. What distinguishes the nursing profession in the 1970s and 1980s is its concern for independence and special professional integrity. This concern leads to controversy in social and professional hierarchies, where not only are physicians generally seen to be those in charge, but medical and nursing licensing laws have established physicians as the only individuals allowed to engage in the major proportion of therapeutic, and a large proportion of caring, procedures. One must remember that prescription of painkillers and tranquilizers is the prerogative of physicians. Further, the economic realities are such that physicians maintain an independence that is not possessed by nurses. It is easier for physicians to practice on their own than for nurses, and hospitals depend upon physicians for maintaining their census. In addition, the weight of tradition makes physicians the captains of the therapeutic team.

Patients in general recognize this fact. Though they may plead through a physician assistant or nurse for a change in medication, it is only the physician who can authorize a change. To appreciate the force of this, one might imagine a society where free men and women could have access to whatever drug they wished on the open market. One might imagine, as well, that there would be no licensing laws, only certifying exams available to all. The populace could be regularly warned by the federal government that it is best to be treated by individuals who have recently passed a federal certifying examination for anesthesiology, obstetrics, psychiatry, etc. To stand for such an exam, one would not need a particular diploma; R.N.s and M.D.s could try, if they wished, as could chiropractors and naturopaths. Such a world would probably look quite different from the one in which we live. However, there would likely be a number of similarities as well.

Good hospitals would tend to give hospital privileges only to those with established abilities and credentials. Just as people now decide among Christian Science practitioners, chiropractors, incompetent and competent physicians, individuals would be able (in this fantasized world) to do somewhat the same. If they could demand to see recent test scores, rather than know only that an individual passed a licensing exam thirty years ago, things might be better than they are now, with regard to choosing in an informed fashion. Among the differences would be the character of nurse-physician relationships, for nurses would not be restrained from diagnosing and treating simply on the basis that they were not physicians. What they could do, and under what circumstances, would depend on their capacity to convince institutions and individuals of their abilities.

Thus the line between nursing and medicine would become even more obscure. It would be almost impossible to tell the difference between anesthesiologists and nurse anesthetists, obstetricians and midwives, psychiatrists and psychiatric nurses. One would suspect that the more elaborate education of physicians would give them greater capacities to act in complicated therapeutic circumstances; but that would be only a general rule, and there would be many exceptions on both sides. Most talk of clear distinctions between nursing diagnoses and medical diagnoses would slowly vanish. One suspects this, for example, if one examines lists of nursing diagnoses. It is difficult to see in most of them, if in any of them, essential differences from medical diagnoses. "Airway clearance, ineffective"; "Bowel elimination, alteration in: Diarrhea"; "Cardiac output, alteration in, decrease"; or "Fluid volume deficit" can all find their medical equivalents. Diagnoses such as "Coping, ineffective individual" or "Thought processes, alteration in" can be given analogues in the Diagnostic and Statistical Manual of the American Psychiatric Association.[8] Even such taxa as "Spiritual distress (distress of the human spirit)" can probably find an analogue in the endeavors of Jungian psychoanalysis.

My point is that there are no essential differences between the therapeutic commitments of nurses and physicians. There are no essential differences between physicians' and nurses' perceptions of normal functioning, acceptable levels of pain and distress, or the character of good human form and grace. Nor are there differences in scientific presuppositions. Rather, the differences appear to be in the different social roles and powers of nurses and physicians.

When one examines the differences in the approaches of physicians and nurses to coping, curing, and caring, marked differences are found (if at all) only in the social differences between nurses and physicians. As the illustration of the fantasy world suggests, when those artifices of legally enforced social convention are erased, there is likely to be an unbroken spectrum between physicianly and nurselike undertakings.

PHYSICIANS, PATIENTS, AND THE PEOPLE IN BETWEEN: NURSES

Nurses give their care under the scrutiny of two rather powerful individuals: the patient and the physician. The physician wields power in being both *an authority* in health care matters, as well as *in authority* in being able to prescribe drugs and perform essential lifesaving and pain-reducing procedures. Physicians are authorities due to the unequal distribution of knowledge in highly technological societies. Lay individuals, often including nurses, cannot adequately assess the complex claims made by physicians. As Alfred Schutz has argued, this inequality of knowledge, which supports the development of experts in advanced societies, leads to social inequalities that can never be fully set aside.[9] Further, as already indicated, physicians are put *in authority* by various societal constraints on individual conduct, including the acquisition of many drugs.[10]

Patients, on the other hand, in a secular pluralist society such as ours, are the sources of authority for health care.[11] It is they who decide what they will allow to be done to them. One might think here of the holding of the Kansas Supreme Court in 1960 in *Natanson v. Kline*: "Anglo-American law starts with the premise of thoroughgoing self determination. It follows that each man is considered to be a master of his own body, and he may, if he be of sound mind, expressly prohibit the performance of life-saving surgery . . ."[12] Or one might better refer to the holding of the United States Court of Appeals in *Canterbury v. Spence*, which set aside the professional standard for disclosure in holding that "the patient's right of self-decision shapes the boundaries of the duty to reveal."[13] This law bearing on medicine reflects a growing appreciation of individuals as the source of authority generally. One might think here of Justice Brandeis's famous dissent in the Olmstead case: "The makers of our Constitution . . . sought to protect Americans in their beliefs, their thoughts, their emotions and their sensations. They conferred, as against the Government, the right to be let alone—the most comprehensive of rights and the right most valued by civilized men."[14] Brandeis's dissent is developed in a dissent by Justice Burger in *In re President and Directors of Georgetown College*: "Nothing in this utterance suggests that Justice Brandeis thought an individual possessed these rights only as to *sensible* beliefs, *valid* thoughts, *reasonable* emotions, or *well-founded* sensations. I suggest he intended to include a great many foolish, unreasonable and even absurd ideas which do not conform, such as refusing medical treatment even at great risk."[15] In short, though patients are often disabled by disease or ignorance, they are clearly recognized as a source of authority for health care. They join as co-equals with physicians in authorizing therapeutic endeavors.

Nurses are caught between physicians, on the one hand, who are authorities regarding scientific and technological knowledge, and are *in authority*, and patients on the other hand, who give authority for health care endeavors. Nurses are often placed, as a result, in ambiguous circumstances regarding which side is authorizing them to do what. Even troubling cases, such as the Tuma case, can be seen in this light. Did Tuma need the authority of a physician to offer therapeutic alternatives, or is it sufficient that she is authorized by the patient? Since the nurse is neither simply the agent of the patient nor the physician, but is treated as the agent of both, the conflicts can be deep and intractable. This ambiguity appears in part to underlie the holding of the Supreme Court of Idaho in the Tuma case. The Court recognized the unclarity regarding what would or would not count as unprofessional conduct, and in doing so acknowledged the ambiguity of the position of nurses.[16]

How one resolves this question will depend upon contrasting views of the proper social structure for the delivery of health care. The more the nurse is seen as the physician's assistant, the more she will be expected to be loyal to the physician's plan of treatment and to consult with authority before providing advice on her own. Such is *not* a morally implausible structure. To carry out well-coordinated projects, participants must give the benefit of the doubt to those they acknowledge to be in authority. Social structures presume that the burden of proof is upon the individual who would depart from the group's objectives. It is not implausible to conceive of the physician as the central arbiter of authority on the side of the health professions. Such, at least, is the case if nurses are willing to accept this model as physician assistants do. However, nurses have rejected this model and seek to be (in part) co-equal with physicians. The result is the tension and unclarity that the Tuma case presents. Such unclarity has led nursing to attempt to discover a conceptual and scientific integrity to justify the independence sought by nurses in the health care hierarchy.[17] Yet, as the foregoing arguments suggest, such a goal is likely to be ephemeral. One will not discover a conceptually unique core to nursing.

This will not divest nursing of its importance, and nurses will fill health care niches where there is no strong competition from physicians. Because of the time available to physicians and to nurses to engage in caring endeavors, nurses will (in general) appear to be somewhat different from physicians in their "investments" in these activities. In part, this will be due to differences in time allotments to particular tasks by physicians and, in part, to the differences in social perquisites and powers. One will be able to identify, along a shifting and uneven border, the boundaries between what nurses and physicians do. It will often (if not usually) be an artificial border—somewhat like walking across the border between the United States and Canada. There will be no startling differences, though the law will have established a boundary.

Given all the foregoing reflections, what can one say about the character of physician-nurse relationships in care of patients? First, one must recognize that the nurse-physician relationship bears only indirectly upon the nature of the health care giver-patient relationship. Even if the former were authoritarian, on the model of physicians being "captains of the ship," it need not follow that the giver-patient relationship must be paternalistic. A physician who employs physician assistants might well instruct them to behave toward patients in a nonpaternalistic fashion. Indeed, the physician may agree with patients, that only the physician and patient will discuss treatment alternatives, and that the physician assistant will never assume that prerogative. Moreover, they might decide that the caring and aid in coping that physician assistants would offer patients will only be the kind agreed to by the patient with the physician. In short, one can fashion a picture of health care delivery in which physician assistants have no independent role and act simply as agents of physicians. One would still have a physician-patient relationship not characterized by paternalism, but by open and candid discussion and nonpaternalistic resolution of issues of mutual concern. The patient and the physician might be seen as two generals, meeting and discussing common battle plans under circumstances where each agrees to ignore unsolicited remarks by junior officers.

Though, in many areas of medicine, such is likely to be the character of physician-nurse relationships in encounters with patients, it is being replaced by models in which nurses and physicians are seen as partners in health care. In actual circumstances, the character of that partnership is likely to be determined by the capacities and areas of expertise of the physicians and nurses. Our fantasy, involving abandonment of restraints, should be taken as instructive here. One will not know who is better at caring for or aiding patients in coping with their diseases, within a particular health care team, until one examines the capacity of the members. It may be the case that nurse members of the team will have more time and skill at their disposal to act as care-givers; other circumstances may allow certain health care providers to assume, for particular patients, the role of supportive father or mother figure. It is unlikely that one will be able to determine, *a priori*, in terms of whether the individuals possess an R.N. or an M.D., whether the nurse or the physician will be better at such a task.

I do not deny that one is likely to find interesting sociological facts regarding proclivities and abilities of male versus female nurses, female versus male psychiatrists, and male versus female physicians. However, such differences in (say) reassuring patients and aiding them in coping are likely to be the result of cultural expectations and conditions as much as the result of nursing and medicine encompassing slightly different bodies of skill or expertise. I am arguing, rather, that the most important differences will depend on individuals and their agreements, as well as the legal constraints imposed by society on nurses and physicians in treating and diagnosing the problems of patients. What people will agree to, and what society will *allow* people to agree to do, will be the most determinative ways in which physicians, nurses, and patients deport themselves in the various theaters of health care.

Physicians, Patients—and Nurses

COPING, CURING, AND CARING:
THE ROLE OF FREE MEN AND WOMEN

One characteristic of health care giver-patient relationships in the United States is the major emphasis upon the rights of patients to determine their own destinies. I have indicated the steps toward acknowledging patients as the masters of their bodies, the first of which is recognition of patients' rights not to be touched or treated without their permission. (Here, generally, the law on health care reflects the law with regard to civil and criminal battery.) Unauthorized touching of another's person is an indignity, which is to be forbidden.[18] This came into the law in America (bearing on medicine) in a famous holding of Justice Cardozo in *Schloendorff* v. *Society of New York Hospital*: "Every human being of adult years and sound mind has a right to determine what shall be done with his own body; and a surgeon who performs an operation without his patient's consent commits an assault, for which he is liable in damages."[19]

This recognition of the right of self-determination has been augmented by acknowledgment of the right of individuals to enter into agreements with other consenting individuals for forms of health care that might be disapproved by many elements of society. Here one thinks of landmark decisions regarding rights to access to contraceptives and contraceptive information, which developed from the Supreme Court ruling in *Griswold* v. *Connecticut*.[20] *Roe* v. *Wade* took this yet further in establishing the right of physicians and patients to agree to the performance of an abortion.[21] However, the Griswold ruling opened the way not only for physicians, but also for nurses and others, to provide contraceptive information to all who wish it. In fact, the *Roe* v. *Wade* decision does not preclude development of a profession of nurseabortionists who would presumably have the same rights as physicians in providing abortions.

What I am trying to emphasize here are the major shifts toward acknowledging individuals, men and women, as the masters of their destinies and the source of institutional authority. The answer to "Whose life is it, anyway?" is "Yours and mine." With that answer comes the responsibility to fashion, with as much forethought as we can, modes of relationships that will allow us to save as many values, and avoid as many harms, as we are able. One must remember that the health care professions have developed to aid individuals in coping with the blind forces of nature, which often are at odds with human purposes, human loves, and human hopes. They are, in the end, the forces that will disable most of us with illness and disease, and will in the end kill us all.

The holdings of the Supreme Court in *Griswold* v. *Connecticut* and *Roe* v. *Wade* indicate the major advances that humans have made in controlling the forces of human biology—here our reproductive functions, which are often at odds with our social obligations and best-laid plans. However, the contributions made by effective, cheap, easily available contraception and low-risk abortion are but some of the many contributions made by health care to our abilities to cope with nature generally, and with our biological nature in particular. The availability of immunizations, antibiotics, surgery, mood-altering and pain-killing drugs, modes of behavioral therapy, and prosthetic organs have contributed, in a revolutionary fashion, to our abilities to cope with the limitations of human biology and to care for individuals who are disabled and injured by illness or accident.

Health care embraces a cluster of institutionalized responses to our finitude. It involves modes of altering and reshaping human nature, as well as aiding us to live with its limitations. Health care, because it deals with finite individuals with often infinite hopes, involves the context of tragedy: hopes are always, in the end, circumscribed and limited, and often crushed. Because health care is directed to free men and women, it involves the moral obligations to gain their consent in common endeavors.

It is here, I think, that it is best to place the change in relations of physicians and nurses to patients. Whether it is better or worse for patients to have nurses function as co-partners in the health care team is likely to be an issue that can be distinguished, if not separated, from two other issues: the role that nurses are *willing* to play and the roles that patients *wish* nurses and physicians to play. These two roles are as important as the first. In fact, it is the issue of the role that nurses wish to play that, as much as anything else, has been the motor for recent changes in the character of the nursing profession. However, it is the last issue, *what patients want*, that should be as determinative as the wishes of nurses and physicians.

Richard M.
Zaner

5. "How the Hell Did I Get Here?" Reflections on Being a Patient

I came across the title of this address while researching what it's like to experience your own kidneys as failed, then having to rely on hemodialysis to keep the impurities in your blood from killing you.[1] The words are those of Lee Foster, one of the fortunate few who is able to sustain self-dialysis at home.[2] The results of those reflections, "Chance and Morality," appeared in the book edited by Victor Kestenbaum, *The Humanity of the Ill*, along with a number of other insightful essays. Two of these, and the inquiries which led to my contribution, are of immediate relevance to the theme I was asked to address for this conference. I want to give merely a brief indication of those two studies, by Mary Rawlinson and Edmund D. Pellegrino, as a way of initiating my present inquiry.

Mary Rawlinson gives four key ways in which illness compromises our ordinary experience.[3] First, space and time, as ordinarily experienced, become transformed— one's sight and reach constrict. For instance, one's body is no longer the silent means for acting, walking, talking, reaching, seeing, hearing, etc., but becomes prominent. When my eyes hurt, I become aware of my embodied seeing; when my breathing becomes labored, I am forced to an awareness of it quite unlike my ordinary experience.

Second, illness "confounds our capacity to expect" (p. 75), in that the continuity of daily life and its concerns are disrupted, plans and prospects are compromised or delayed—perhaps irreversibly obstructed.

Third, illness is not sought out (except in pathological conduct), but "happens"; it befalls me unbidden. "Sickness never constitutes a value in itself which one might appropriately cultivate. One falls ill" (p. 76), and the consequent prominence of my pain, my aches, my inabilities to do as before, seems thereby to limit my capacity to conduct my life, to be in charge of myself and my affairs. Instead, I find I have to comply with the demands of my ailing body. Illness has its own demands, its own time, its own constraints, and lies beyond my control—and often my direct awareness or knowledge.

Fourth, "illness distorts our ordinary relations with others insofar as it debilitates, humiliates, and isolates" (p. 76). I can no longer "do for myself," as I formerly did, and am "at the mercy of others to regulate, manipulate, investigate, and, perhaps, restore those failing capacities" (p. 77). Illness thus invariably involves some degree of "surrender of one's autonomy and integrity," because this is necessary for the hoped-for restoration of failed capacities (p. 77).

Pellegrino's reflections in "Being Ill and Being Healed,"[4] intended to provide the ground for a more appropriate "medical morality" in our technological times, agree very much with Rawlinson's. Unlike our less technologically sophisticated forebears, we modern persons find illness a far more "insistently painful experience," "more terrifying, more disabling"—a veritable "ontological assault" on our humanly defining characteristics (pp. 157–58). Living in a universe no longer constituted as a cosmos (whether thought to be malignant, benign, indifferent, or beneficent), illness is for modern man an "undesired, unsought, capricious irruption," an "absurdity," because it seems ultimately unaccountable and undeserved (p. 158).

For modern man, then, illness is an assault on what is understood to be his humanity, in five distinct ways. First, it ruptures the ordinarily experienced intimacy of human life, whether by bringing the afflicted body "to center stage" or by striking at the psyche or spirit in emotional or mental distress. The usual unity of human life is breeched. Second, illness "erodes the image we have constructed over the years, often painfully, of ourselves and our world" (p. 158). At times, this is even threatened with irreversible compromise or total collapse.

Third, in illness "we lose most of the freedom we ordinarily associate with being able to act as a fully human person" (p. 159). Most often, we do not understand what's happened to us, how it can be cured (if at all), what futures are in store for us, or even whether those who profess to heal really can do so.

Fourth, we become unusually reliant on other persons—in a relationship, however, which is profoundly unequal: "for the healer professes to possess precisely what the patient lacks—the knowledge and power to heal" (p. 159). With this, finally, we are uniquely diminished, unlike any other modality of deprivation (e.g., poverty, imprisonment). "In no other deprivation is the dissolution of the person so intimate that it impairs the capacity to deal with all other deprivations" (p. 159).

On Being a Patient

Adjusting for respective angles of vision and the dictates of respectively preoccupying themes, I had come up with very much these same basic characteristics in studying kidney disease and hemodialysis. Yet a number of puzzles still remain, and these seem especially pertinent for grappling with the issue I was asked to address here: the patient *in relation to* the health professionals.

Surely, one might say, it is unquestionably essential for a physician or nurse to understand that illness or injury results in more or less damage to a person's autonomy, integrity, self-image, and relatedness to other people. Failure to understand this in the most practical ways could result in inappropriate medical or nursing conduct, and this could be additionally damaging to the patient. But this concerns the professionals in relation to the patient, and we are now asked to consider this relationship from the other end. Just as going from here to there is not at all the same as going from there to here, so must the present theme oblige us to reconsider this business of being ill from the patient's actual perspective, not from that of the health care providers—not even from that of an especially sensitive third party. Our task is something different; and even if this is a slight difference, it could make *all* the difference.

To attain this perspective, there is nothing to do but consult patients themselves—ourselves included (as should be obvious). "Them," the patients, are "us." Patients must be allowed to speak, then—ourselves included. However, several caveats seem in order.

First, our task is not to "put ourselves in the place of patients," to empathize (even though this surely has a significant place) with "them." Rather we need, on the one hand, to listen to patients and to engage in active remembering of ourselves as ill or injured. Second, we must be wary of the too-easy presumption that other patients are like ourselves, or—similarly—to presume that those for whom words come easily say all there is to say about illness. To correct for these tendencies, clinical experience seems centrally helpful, so long as one can resist the temptation to view patients solely through the eyes and words of clinicians.

In this effort, we can be greatly helped by using Robert Hardy's fascinating compilation of interviews with some sixty different, and differently afflicted, patients.[5] Published with the lay-it-all-out title, *Sick: How People Feel about Being Sick and What They Think of Those Who Care for Them*, Hardy simply allowed these people to talk, which they do—willingly and copiously—about their pains, anxieties, suffering, complaints, their doctors and nurses and hospitals and lawyers and insurance companies.

Each of these stories constitutes a sort of clinical pathological conference (CPC)—quite unlike the more familiar medical sort, however. For these are, as Hardy remarks, "conducted in homes, in doctors' waiting rooms, in bars, at cocktail parties, in private corners and all the places former patients gather to talk about being sick" (p. xi). Here, the doctor or nurse is almost never invited, and, if known to be present, alters the CPC in basic ways.

One patient, a 40-year-old woman, seeking to have a "tuck"—and got far more grief than she'd bargained for—says at one point:

You have to trust these people, the physicians, like you do God. You're all in their hands, and if they don't take care of you, who's going to? It's God and them. It is really a responsibility and I think a doctor should have a little more dedication to the patient. I took him at his word . . . I trusted him not to let an inexperienced person mess up my life [p. 40].

Which, of course, is just what happened: an assistant was allowed to do the left side of her abdomen, and the panniculectomy was fouled up.

Up to that point, she was, like most patients, quite submissive, obedient, and cooperative. She believed, as do most of us, that it is essential to maintain this cooperative relationship—if for nothing else, for your own protection—precisely in view of what Pellegrino pointed out: the unequal relationship which puts power on the side of the physician.

From the patient's perspective, then, the uncommon dependency on physicians may be, and often is, textured by the patient's clear perception that the physician is indeed in charge, and able to do what the patient cannot do, and may not even want done. "It's God and them," and her point seems to be that a good part of patient compliance is based on wanting to stay on the good side of the care providers—to protect yourself. To the head surgeon's glib remark, "Really, you don't look that bad," she replied: "If I wore a girdle, I didn't look that bad before I came to you, and for $2,000 you're supposed to make me look better." She concluded: "The next operation is on him" (p. 43).

At times, the sort of attitude this woman exhibited at the beginning of her experience—compliance, trust, etc.—can get patients in real trouble. Oddly, even though many patients may know this in advance, they are haphazard in the way they select doctors and in the way they "stick" with them even after bad experiences. For instance, one couple, seeking a fertility test, reported that "just by asking around, we got onto another doctor" (p. 105). Another patient, told that she should consult a gynecologist, said: "I worked on OB at the hospital as a unit clerk and know some of the specialists but I really can't tell you why I settled on Dr. Smith" (p. 108). This was no minor thing, either: she wanted to be sterilized, and "stayed" with Dr. Smith, even though he subsequently performed a laparoscopy (apparently for no other reason than that the hospital had just acquired such an instrument and he thought he might check out his work). She developed kidney disease—about which risk she had not been informed—and to top it all off, she got pregnant (pp. 109–10). She sued Dr. Smith, but only after he had the audacity to charge her for the botched surgery, although he had said he wasn't going to charge her. Only then did she see a lawyer.

These remarks, and others like them, demonstrate how patients are remarkably resilient and forgiving— published statistics to the contrary notwithstanding. These (and other) patients seem reluctant to pursue legal redress, even where it may not be unreasonable. Unexpectedly, this woman, like so many others, was able to understand that physicians are human, too; that they make mistakes; and that only at times are they culpable. Often, what's important for these patients seems not the mistakes, but the willingness (or unwillingness) of the physician to own up to a mistake and be ready to make amends in some reasonable and caring way (p. 114).

Thus—though vulnerable, compromised, weakened, and subservient—patients are nonetheless uncommonly prepared and able to understand, and forgive. At the same time, they not unreasonably expect physicians and nurses to show their own humanity, not only in their mistakes but in their subsequent conduct as well.

To become ill and be hospitalized is to enter into a forbidding and foreign environment. One is surrounded by other persons who, invariably, are not fully known, although some may know each other, and what they are doing, but health professionals do not always try—or succeed even if they try—to tell patients what's going on with them. To undergo hospitalization is a form of culture shock. It is to find oneself, in Alfred Schutz's idiom, a "stranger,"[6] however temporary it may be.

Not only have hospitals been recognized as forbidding places sociologically but also architecturally, designed more to enhance than to ameliorate this foreignness. The people who populate them—other patients, administrative personnel, nursing staff and aides, clerks, volunteers, food processors, physicians and house staff—as well as their artifacts—are strange. Moreover, patients are stripped of familiar things (clothes, possessions) and made to put on nondescript gowns that permit ready access to their bodies—to disclose their intimate details of personal life to whoever takes their history, to expose their bodies in the most intimate and humiliating postures, for strangers to poke and prod, swab and stick, palpate and feel—in a continuous daily round. To be a patient requires remarkable patience.

Thus it is hardly surprising that many patients, even to themselves, seem out of place—beyond what their illnesses may have brought about. As one patient pointed out, "people are timid around doctors" (*Sick,* p. 92). Culture shock can only be intensified by the debilitating effects of illness itself. For instance, a young man with ulcerative colitis stated that the "ileostomy is hardly any hassle at all, once I got used to it, but it's just the emotional part, losing a part of your body which you have had all of your life" (*Sick,* p. 337). Another patient reported that his real problem in being hospitalized (with gall bladder attack) was

not having information. I was being called upon to make a decision at a time when, first of all, I had no awareness

Richard M. Zaner

of what the lab reports would show, if anything . . .
although my physician indicated that my problem was a
gall bladder problem, I was not sure that he had very
much confirming evidence in terms of the x-rays and lab
work, since neither was available or at least had not been
reported to me at that time [*Sick*, p. 246].

The strangeness of what is happening to a patient can
itself present critical problems. A judge, for instance,
who developed diabetes, emphasized that "there are lots
of feelings that are hard to put into words, especially if
you've never had the feeling before. I had to explain
things to my doctor which were a brand new experience
to me, and I had nothing to compare it to" (*Sick*, p. 236).
The dimensions of the alien multiply and complicate not
only patient life but treatment as well.

On the other hand, the strange can at times be made
somewhat comfortable, can more readily be reckoned
with, and confidence can be restored or maintained. As a
heart attack victim reported, "we were like a team and
this was a campaign. I was a member of the team. I was
the cause of all the trouble but I was also a member of the
team. We were holding hands" (*Sick*, p. 209). A patient
with lung cancer emphasized: "When the doctor told me
I had this tumor, frankly, it alarmed me, but he did it in
such a way that left me with a feeling of confidence. He
was outright and open about it" (*Sick*, p. 9).

Yet the sense of strangeness and being unable to
reckon with things, to take one's bearings, when wors-
ened by lack of information, is commonly one of the
clearest memories of patients. Hearing a patient com-
plain that her doctors didn't "tell me a darn thing," a
woman stressed: "I felt sure they wouldn't. I don't think
they do it on purpose. I just think they take their job so
for granted that they do a good job but they fail to inform
a person. They don't realize we are so ignorant as to what

we are paying for" (*Sick*, p. 43). And as the mother of an asthmatic boy said: "Doctors do not tell you all of the things to look for. It could be that they don't have time but then there's something terribly wrong with our society. They should have time" (*Sick*, p. 60).

What becomes pretty obvious is that many patients have compelling difficulties in their efforts, their desires, to find out what's going on with them. Possibly, some fear being regarded as too pushy, as presumptuous; others may be apprehensive about being insulting. However that may be, hospitals are rarely places which encourage persistent questions from patients. They are busy places; people are busy; and things are always serious. Questions interrupt nurses and physicians in their daily round of activities, especially (it is said) in their care of other patients. Questions may thus appear selfish, and patients do not want to appear presumptuous, insulting, or selfish—in hospitals no less than in other settings in life.

Furthermore, patients aren't in a good position to question those who take care and have control over them; they can often not evaluate what's being done to them, nor judge whether treatments are appropriate. Being ill, as Rawlinson and Pellegrino say, severely compromises this even more. Open and direct communication, though difficult enough in hospitals, can be further compromised: some patients do not know how to talk to nurses and doctors; others may not want to do so (at a particular time, or at all); and some are content to act out the sick role as they believe they are expected (and perhaps even encouraged) to do by doctors and nurses. A premium is placed, after all, on the "good patient," who is compliant, cooperative, quiet, etc.

Learning that he had diabetes, the judge pointedly remarked:

If you can't communicate and you can't understand your disease, then you don't have any confidence in the medical help you are getting. The better the doctor explains to you, the better position you're in to abide by what he wants you to do. . . . If you don't get up some relationship with your doctor, then you can't tell him what's wrong with you. . . . So, if you can't communicate back and forth, and explain to him what's bothering you, how can he help you? [*Sick,* p. 236].

The mother of a partially sighted child stated that if you have a good mind,

you want your doctor to understand that. . . . But people are too timid around doctors. . . . They have become superhuman because of the way people treat them. Until you've been around doctors as friends you don't realize that they have fears, too. But . . . they sense how timid you are and that makes them more overpowering. They've got an edge on you. . . . Somehow if doctors could just sense how much hold they have over a person's feelings . . . [*Sick,* pp. 89, 92].

To review thus far: as patients view the matter, the inequality of the patient-professional relationship is no mystery but, while they are sick, a daily reality to be contended with. This is true even though it presents patients with one more agonizing issue. In ordinary life, such inequalities are of course common, as is the variety of ways that are socially available to us to deal with them. When one is sick, however, inequality is qualitatively different, and ways of dealing with it are not ready to hand. As one patient bluntly put it, "You have to trust these people, the physicians"; but also, of course, the nurses, lab technicians, researchers, dieticians, administrators, and the rest.

On Being a Patient

And trust them patients do—to the point that not only are physicians selected in haphazard ways, but patients very often stick with them even when mistakes are made, or a physician has become unable to be of further help. As a patient says, "If they don't take care of you, who's going to?"

In a certain sense, this may be understandable. Nobody likes to dwell on sickness; most patients simply don't think of health professionals or hospitals or clinics unless it has become necessary (often, at crisis times). This lack of concern about health professionals and institutions can lead to haphazard selection when unforeseen illness occurs and treatment is urgently needed. Obviously, there are other factors at work here.

Beyond the strangeness of the settings of health care, patients undergo numerous other reinforcements of the unfamiliar: the unknowns of their condition, the difficulties this implies for understanding and reckoning with what information is obtained (if any), and the sometimes compelling problems of trying to talk about oneself and one's feelings when these are new and unfamiliar.

Finally, patients suffer from difficulties of asking for help or information from those who are seen to be "overpowering" and " in charge" of them, their bodies, and their possible futures. To develop the trust and confidence necessary for getting well, patients understand the need to establish a good relationship with their nurses and physicians; yet, doing just that presents them (or many of them) with painful problems. In a society in which relationships among strangers predominate, in which "being a neighbor" has become rare, communication tends to be designed more for temporary ease of social passage than for in-depth disclosures. Being sick and in a hospital in such a society complicates this more.

These roughly drawn categories require considerable refinement if these patients' words are to be useful. In an unpublished reflection on his experiences in collecting these stories, Hardy suggests, but does not elaborate on, two persistent themes of these stories: sick people "want to *know* and they want to know that the people who are taking care of them *really* care."[7] Indeed, reading these stories, or listening to patients talk about their experiences, we are surprised to learn how much they know about rare diseases, as well as complex medical or surgical procedures to deal with their conditions. Even more remarkable, patients are frequently fascinated and intrigued by the wild growths, bumps, gurgles, bulges, spasms and jerks their bodies display and the procedures and tests they go through to have them diagnosed and treated. They often report how "interesting" it was to be prepared for surgery; to have an angiogram or vasectomy; to be radiated at just the right spot for cancer; to learn what various tubes, running in and out of one's body, are for; and even to find out what happened during coronary bypass surgery.

Patients *want* to know. The physician, Robert S. Mendelsohn, who wrote the Introduction to Hardy's book, was so impressed by this that he was moved to emphasize: "A remarkable finding of these interviews is the consistently profound base of information patients manifest about their condition . . . patients are aware of the major aspects as well as the subtleties of causation, diagnosis, treatment alternatives and predictions of outcomes" (*Sick*, pp. vii–viii). They also show unexpected appreciation of the dilemmas, successes, failures, and mistakes of clinical practice—whether they are then moved to forgiveness, apology, or condemnation. Mendelsohn thinks the message is loud and clear: "Stop talking down to your patients; stop patronizing them as if they were children or stupid or retarded or all three" (*Sick*, p. viii).

Patients want to *know*—and often succeed in finding out; and are fascinated, despite the reticence or reluctance or silence of physicians and nurses. In a way, I think, to be a patient is to be constantly *on the alert*, to the extent and in whatever ways are possible, for any "news" about themselves. A patient with emphysema and pneumonia, who was told "very little" about his problem, noted how acutely alert he became to any talk: "I got provoked with my doctor. He was talking with a resident physician who makes rounds with him, a young doctor, and I heard him tell that doctor I've only got 16 percent and he didn't see how I could do as well as I did. . . . Well, it made me mad and I was very depressed" (*Sick*, p. 53). He thought that maybe he was wrong to feel so good—or else that he would "show" that doctor!

Earlier in his illness, he noted that while he was still in the ICU, "I don't guess the doctors knew I could hear them, but I heard them talking and they were going to do a tracheotomy. I remember that. I was in there three weeks and, oh, it was just like being in a cell" (*Sick*, p. 49). One patient I have seen went so far as to interpret an intern's silence (or inability to discuss his condition with him) as "bad news," figuring—as he later said—"that if only the 'big cheese' could tell me what was wrong, it must be bad news."

This wanting to know must be given its full due. In strange environments, ailing, and not fully understanding why, or what the immediate future will bring; with pain and anxiety demanding and capturing your attention; facing strangers who propose and carry out intrusions into your body, with faces grave and committed to crisis, a coronary patient reports that "you really grasp at the things which are encouraging and anything that intimates you've really got something wrong with you, you grab onto that, too, so you have two hands full of straw" (*Sick,* p. 223).

In alien territory, a person quite naturally reconnoiters the terrain, seeks familiar or interpretable signs by which to locate and situate himself, to know what to reckon with and what to hold by, as Ortega y Gasset often expressed it. This natural response to finding oneself in unfamiliar regions—which is made acute by being sick, distressed, or injured—is another clear and commanding reminder of how important it is for the patient to know and to understand, however this need may be expressed and whether expressed well, poorly, or even silently. One seeks to know, but this may not be recognized by physicians and nurses, who are more familiar with and accustomed to the hospital environs. Indeed, precisely what they have come to take for granted—not simply about diseases and medical or surgical regimens, but more: the complex of folkways, mores, rules, regulations, habits, customs, etiquette, fashions, multiple corridors, and things and people that populate health care institutions—is precisely what the patient cannot take for granted yet must reckon with. Sociologically, the patient is a special kind of "stranger" in Schutz's meaning.

In these terms, it is hardly surprising—is in fact to be expected—that the patient's preoccupation in such institutions is a seeking to know, which at times will construe the most innocuous and unrelated gestures, words, gossip, objects, and circumstances as imbued with deep meaning, whether "dire" and "foreboding" or "encouraging" and "hopeful." As Eric Cassell has emphasized, suffering, as distinct from pain, is a threat to a patient's sense of self. A prominent form of suffering, indeed, is not knowing why one hurts, or the source of the pain, or its significance for "what's going on" with a patient.[8] Not disclosing such information means that the patient is *abandoned*, having to guess at what's going on—abandoned even to haphazard interpretation of recondite signs.

Given all these considerations—the remarkable understanding people characteristically have about their own and their loved ones' sicknesses, and how we all, in any case, interpret our circumstances, seeking and finding meaning therein (whether well or poorly), so that we can know what to hold by and to reckon with—it would appear that something very like a norm of conduct by health professionals not only follows but seems demanded by afflicted persons from the sheer "facticity" of their being human and afflicted. Patients want and seek to know, and in the interest of proper and appropriate dealing with them, the norm that obliges that accurate, adequate, and understandable information be promptly and continuously given to them seems unquestionably demanded.

Any *departure* from open and continuous sharing of information, which is intelligible and understandable to patients, would seem, just as clearly, in need of sound rationale and justification. However, it seems equally true that any purported rationale for withholding information that is vital to allow patients honestly to orient themselves must, in the first place, be discussed with patients.

Evidence shows that patients are capable of understanding and grappling with their conditions far better than had been thought. It is also unmistakably the case that, as the diabetic judge put it, "if you can't communicate and you can't understand your disease, then you don't have any confidence in the medical help you're getting. The better the doctor explains to you, the better position you're in to abide by what he wants you to do" (*Sick*, p. 236). Or, as the mother of the child with congenital cataracts says, "you love to run into a doctor who is not condescending. If you feel like your mind is good too, you want your doctor to understand that" (*Sick*, p. 89). A knowledgeable patient is not only more likely to be cooperative, but also more likely to benefit from what health professionals can offer.

Hardy emphasizes that patients want to know, and equally that they want to know that those who take care of them *really* care.

Rawlinson, Pellegrino, Cassell, and others have helped us understand the deeper dimensions of being ill, emotionally or mentally distressed, and injured or handicapped. In a sense, it is precisely because of these dimensions of being afflicted that, Hardy remarks, "people need caring, empathetic health professionals to relieve the stark terror of not knowing what is going to happen to them" ("My Turn"). This is especially true when the news is "bad." Too often, nurses and physicians tend to retreat from being bearers of bad news. Although we no longer put such messengers to death, as was done in certain ancient cultures, the stigma of bearing bad news remains for many people. But retreating from telling this to patients, or attempting to mute its sting, may be quite ineffective: patients' knowledge or awareness of themselves often confutes such efforts, which in any case may be unconscious (or partially conscious) self-protective devices of the health professionals. More importantly, every patient's affliction means crucial diminishment (if only temporary), possible loss and compromise, perhaps even devastation or death. To compound this evident suffering with the additional terror and suffering of *not knowing* seems plainly too much.

This "too much," moreover, bespeaks a fundamental moral dimension inherent to patients' relations to health professionals: the appeal to others not merely to diagnose, test, treat, and prognose, but *to care* for them.

The commonly coupled terms, "health care," which too often is bureaucratized into the far different (and possibly immoral) "health management," is an ineluctably moral notion at the heart of medicine, in the broadest sense. This is as evident from patients' dismay, humiliation, and anger at not being told about their conditions (and thus not being respected, "cared for") as it is in their praise and gratitude when they have been treated with respect vis-à-vis their wanting, and ability, to understand.

A retired college English professor in her middle 70s, speaking about the treatment her extremely ill sister received (or failed to receive) and their frustrations in obtaining medical help, concluded in exasperation: "It is a totally helpless feeling, so frustrating and disgusting. You get to thinking, 'What is this thing of medical training doing for training doctors to be interested in their patients or in building a profession?' I think it's serious. . . . What is the problem?" (*Sick*, p. 292).

Another critic reports losing confidence in her family physician simply because he hadn't kept current with new developments and thereby created additional problems for her (*Sick*, p. 285). On the other hand, a patient who suffered a severe gall bladder attack, though he was "put off" by his physicians' giving so little information, reports that he "had very good feelings" about the nurses because of "their ability to deal with members of my family and with me and their response, the care with which they dealt with me as a patient. They dealt with me more as a person than a patient" (*Sick*, p. 247).

A truck driver, irritated by never being allowed to say anything to the doctor (who treated him in his office), by the rush and the lack of time, said: "You go to the doctor's office and you sit for about an hour past your appointment and then you get up and go sit in the examinin' room or the shot room for another 15 to 20 minutes. . . . This irritates me. In the old days, I believe that people entered the doctor profession out of compassion and caring for other people. But not one person in 10 believes that they do today" (*Sick,* p. 186).

Patients want to know that those who care for them really care. To be sick or injured is to experience ourselves as diminished, as afflicted to various degrees, and in precisely those ways which mark us as distinctively human: in our freedom to choose and act, our ability to think and imagine and plan, the intimacy of our relatedness to our own bodies and minds, and our relatedness to other persons. To want to know and to be really cared for, as afflicted, is a uniquely demanding moral phenomenon, invariably presented within a complex and compelling *pathos.*

These wants are most pronounced at the very time when people are most vulnerable, exposed, disrupted, even bewildered—when we are ill, injured, or distressed, and thus not always able to say what we want and need. Moreover, not only are ways of relieving these forms of suffering difficult to come by for most of us, but often are quite low on the current totems of medical and nursing education and practice. They are made further complicated because patients often cannot, or will not, tell physicians and nurses what really troubles them. Patients may be uneasy, leery, or unhappy with the treatments they receive, but commonly are reluctant to say so.

The pathos defining the patient's relation to health professionals is also textured and troubled by the ways in which time and space are socially structured in the settings where treatment is delivered. To try to establish the kind of communication the diabetic judge emphasizes as necessary for effective care, to learn to talk about wholly new, intimate, and strange feelings or pains, takes time—time to allow these feelings and pains to find their proper words, time to allow health providers to know what troubles the patient. In short, patience is required to permit patients to be themselves.

Space, too, is needed. Unfamiliar surroundings need to become familiar enough to allow such conversation, for patients to become somewhat comfortable. The settings of current practice seem rarely designed to provide either time or space.

Most poignantly, to be a patient is to find yourself in the predicament of *having to trust* those who care for you (in a sense, whether you like it or not), even though those who treat you are most often complete strangers. The central moments of being sick—wanting to know, to be cared for, to become well again, being vulnerable and diminished—are rendered deeply problematic, as well as paradoxical, by the fact that this necessary trust or confidence, already difficult by the fact of the illness itself, seems least encouraged by the current educational formats and major organizational health care settings. The very times when you are most intimately exposed are the times when, by the nature of the case, you are obliged to be most trusting. The times and occasions which seem least likely to promote that trust are the times and occasions when this is unavoidably forced on you.

The special pathos of illness and distress is a complex and compelling moral phenomenon.

This brings me to a final set of reflections about patients' relations to nurses and physicians and the institutions of their daily practice and encounter. It is doubtless commonplace to note (as we have had occasion to note) how patients are so centered on themselves. What is obvious, however, can mislead us in nonobvious ways; neither in philosophy nor in medicine can the apparently obvious be unexamined. The following are merely suggestions concerning the unexpected and nonobvious dimensions beneath what is taken for granted.

The patient whose words gave me the title of this address spoke them in an interesting context. Afflicted with endstage renal disease, on hemodialysis at home, he reflected:

Yet sometimes when I'm feeling fine, and the machine is running perfectly, and I've enjoyed my dinner, and the music is good and the book I'm reading is interesting, and our cat is purring around my feet, and (my wife) Leslie is smiling at me, a thought suddenly runs through my head: "How the hell did I get here?" ["Man and Machine," p. 6].

Illness is remarkable and disturbing, for unlike anything else in our lives it *uniquely singles me out as me*, as *this* individual person I am: the bodily pain, the anxiety over future prospects, the way in which my condition occupies (and preoccupies) so many people around me, the way so much has to be reorganized and rescheduled, and the riveting focus of the pain and strange new feelings. How did *I* get here?

In some part, this singular experience has its source in the sheer happenstance of illness: it befalls me without my having wanted or chosen it. To try to find some reason for my having fallen ill, in the end, is to try to find some reason for being myself—for me at all. How did I get singled out for this illness?

In some part, too, this has its source in what is

forcefully demonstrated by it: not only is each of us affected in basic ways that make us human, even more fundamentally it marks each of us as *able to die*, as threatened by and exposed to *not being*. In all I am and was and ever hoped to be, I find myself exposed to not-being, to finality. This is not mere self-centeredness; this is a unique singling out of the individual as the person he or she is through telling glimpses of death, of no longer being that person.

Wanting to know and wanting to be cared for, therefore, are appeals that seek response, wants that need recognition and help: *I* am sick and *I* need help. Not simply this, however, for I need help from *you*. To want care, in this deeply personal sense, is *to want to be this self* in *your* eyes and hands, of this nurse, this doctor—just as trust is a deeply personal wanting to know and be with the nurse and physician as the persons they are.

Illness is thus uniquely dyadic; it uniquely appeals for recognition by persons for persons. This medical dyad, caring and trusting, is thus a profoundly moral phenomenon. The promise of this relationship is that not only may the sick person recover from the illness; more to the point, it *promises the recovery of ourselves*, patients and caregivers, *as persons*. The promise may not be fulfilled; it may be broken, ignored, or not even seen as such (for a variety of reasons, good and bad). But even death, or dying, can provide the occasion for this recovery of ourselves.

Illness may be the mask that death often wears, giving glimpses, perhaps, only of death itself. And if this experience singles you or me out in preparation for the final abandonment, the medical dyad establishes us as bound together in our common humanity. It thus promises the mutual enablement of our lives together. As the cardiac patient said: "I was a member of the team"; that is, patient and nurse and physician had recovered themselves in their communality. In this respect, it seems most appropriate and accurate to understand the patient/physician and patient/nurse relationship as a *covenant* and not as a contract.

Illness—the presence of an afflicted person—seems uniquely capable, as Albert Schweitzer saw, of awakening "a moral sense that is usually dormant but that on special occasions can be brought to the surface."⁹ This "sense" has its meaning in the promise which is presented, of recovering our common humanity by responding to the appeal, to the trust that being cared for evokes.

A 42-year-old coronary bypass patient, a man, said a peculiar thing:

I feel great. I wouldn't take anything for this total experience, wouldn't trade it with anyone. This will sound stupid, I'm sure, but it was one of the best things that happened to me in my whole life, having the heart attack, having the angiogram and having the bypass. It did several things for me in other ways. It brought back what I would consider for myself, not necessarily for others, a new system of values. Many things which I had been overlooking for years now have a great deal of meaning for me. Life itself has more meaning for me, each day, each breath. Things which I had taken for granted for ˙ so many years are important. It really doesn't matter whether a job gets done, or you're late or you're on time because if you don't take each breath, who cares? You're always one breath or one heart beat away from extinction [*Sick,* p. 229].

What I have identified as the singularizing experience of illness comes through in these words. But there is something else here which also is remarkable: gratitude. He is, of course (as is plain in his earlier remarks), grateful to his wife and family for "putting up" with him and sticking by him, to the physicians and surgeons and nurses (for the most part), and to the technologies that made it possible for him to recover. But he is also grateful for his "total experience," for having recovered "new values" and a new sense of priorities—of what is truly important for him.

Other patients' reports are similar about gratitude,[10] as well as their moving experiences (*Sick*, pp. 208, 216–17). Even where this complex sense of gratitude is not overtly or well expressed, most patients are not only willing but eager to talk about their illness experiences, to share them with other persons, while in the hospital or afterward. They are especially eager to share what they have learned with persons who later come down with the same sorts of afflictions.

Although matters become very subtle here, I think something quite significant can be detected in these words. There is a sense—not always fulfilled by any means—of what Albert Schweitzer said so eloquently:

All through the world, there is a special league of those who have known anxiety and physical suffering. A mysterious bond connects those marked by pain. They know the terrible things men can undergo; they know the longing to be free of pain. Those who have been liberated from pain must not think they are now completely free again and can calmly return to life as it was before.[11]

Knowledge of the "terrible things men can undergo" indelibly marks us. Having been sick or injured, we know the pain and the anxiety, and the longing to be free from them, as well as the gratitude we feel toward those who both put up with us and care for and treat us. And, once free from pain and anxiety, we know the profound sense of recovery of our health (to the extent this is possible) and of ourselves.

The fulfillment of the promise, when and insofar as it occurs, is *obligating*. The relief, and the experiential knowledge which is its context, also are obligating, and deeply moral. Just as one who is ill seems ineluctably to present himself or herself as needing our help (the helpless can be the occasion for awakening a moral sense), so is experience of the aftermath of illness marked by gratitude and intimate knowledge.

Having this knowledge, being marked by the gratefulness of recovery, seems to bear a moral meaning that is often undetected and unencouraged. Our good fortune in being enabled, by others, to recover obligates: this good luck which befalls the patient, no less than the illness itself, must not (as Schweitzer says) be taken for granted, its burden muted or forgotten. For now, having been ill and having recovered, patients are obligated to give something in return to others, especially to those who now find themselves marked by pain, anxiety, and suffering and long to be free of them.

The patient's relationship to those who care for him or her, I suggest, is a complex and compelling moral phenomenon: it awakens or calls out an otherwise dormant moral sense, and at the same time relates back to the patient. The one who was cared for, and is now free from pain, must now care for others who need this care. Physicians and nurses who have been patients may well be the best caregivers.

Patients—that is, all of us—no less than physicians and nurses, are engaged in a distinctively moral enterprise: being human, knowing "the terrible things man can un-

On Being a Patient

dergo," and enabling others to bear that burden. The pathos of illness thus evokes another side: the reflexive demand to give something in return for our good fortune in recovering ourselves.

6. Further
Considerations

The title of the conference at which these papers were given was "Coping, Curing, Caring: Patient, Physician, Nurse Relationships." The book has been entitled *Caring, Curing, Coping* because the actual theme of the conference became caring. All the participants, including the two physicians, contend that physicians and nurses are in a common caring profession of which curing is only a part. Thus they reject the implication that physicians cure and nurses care. Further, while they recognize that attempting to cope with illness leads ill people to seek professional care, the goal of this care is to help the patients become capable of caring for themselves.

Having abandoned the curing-caring distinction, none of the participants was able to draw a sharp distinction between the nature of medicine and nursing. Obviously, further consideration needs to be given to distinguishing between physician and nurse in theory and practice if both have the common foundation of caring. All the authors recognize that this common foundation implies that physician, nurse, and technician work together as a team. But further consideration is needed of how these relationships could be developed in actual practice. Certainly this should include considerations of actual team relationships which are effective, and recognize special competencies and consider the rights and values of all involved. Since the authors focus mostly on hospital settings, these considerations should include the relationship of physician and nurse in settings other than hospitals, such as physicians' offices, clinics and other ambulatory care settings.

It certainly should include, as well, recent developments in health care. For example, what effect does the development of nurse practitioners have on the relationships of physicians and nurses? Or, as nurses and technicians become more expert in various areas of health care than physicians, how does this affect the traditional role of physician as team leader?

Although all the authors agree that caring is the common foundation for health care professionals, this common foundation is often not apparent in the day-to-day relationships of physicians, nurses, technicians, and patients. Is this lack of common foundation in practice the result of increased stress on the science and technology of curing, as the panelists suggest? If so, has the recent stress on the biomedical led to two interpretations of the practice of medicine: one as cure and one as care? Or are recent developments in medicine imperceptibly changing the practice of medicine from caring to curing, while many practicing nurses and physicians still articulate their profession to be one of caring? Both cases call for a serious philosophical debate to consider the nature of medical practice. In the second case, a reexamination of health care which incorporates biomedical developments into the caring tradition may be necessary.

All of the panelists agree that the patient has the right

to make the final determination concerning treatment; but they also contend that the patient's involvement should be as part of a team. Recently, health care workers have become more concerned about patient rights. Unfortunately, this concern seems a response more to judicial decisions than moral considerations. The panelists, while not denying the importance of legal considerations, contend that patient rights ought to be primarily a moral concern. Further, they warn against limiting moral considerations to rights. Also, they point out that, in any medical decision and patient care, the rights and values of all health care workers, as well as those of the patient, must be considered. How can the rights of all involved be recognized and the care of the patient be focal, rather than medical practice focusing on securing rights and avoiding the consequences of their neglect?

All the panelists agree that patients have the right to know the truth concerning their illness, their treatment, and their prognosis. But having the right to know does not necessarily imply that one *ought* to be told. What if a patient does not want to know? What if the patient is incapable of understanding? Should the physician share his doubts and uncertainties with the patient? How do health care workers tell the truth when comprehension by the patient requires that the patient first come to an adequate level of self-understanding? How does the health care worker convey the truth to a patient who may not grasp its meaning if the truth is stated technically, or nontechnically but from a medical perspective? Put differently, how can health care workers, who think and speak from a medical perspective, translate the meaning of an illness and alternative treatments in terms of the implications for a patient's way of living? Does this need for translation imply a more humanistic education than most health care workers receive?

Further Considerations

Although the panelists see from a common perspective, each panelist suggests issues that need further consideration. That is not to say that other panelists do not treat these issues in a significant way, but that a particular panelist focuses our attention on an issue in a way that requires further consideration.

Pellegrino forces us to face the distinction between curing and caring and its implications for medical practice. He uses cure "in a radical sense—to refer to the eradication of the cause of an illness or disease, to the radical interruption, and reversal of the natural history of the disorder."

Do most practicing physicians understand curing in this radical way? If not, how do they distinguish cure from care? Does the attempt to found a more adequate ethic for physicians require a curing model or a caring model for medicine? Is the contest for an adequate basis for the relationship of physician and patient only between a curing and a caring relationship?

Does the "professional" model, which Engelhardt discusses, need to be considered? If so, is this model primarily concerned with the physician's well-being, considered from the perspective of either curing or caring? How can a professional ethic, adequate for our pluralistic society, treat the problem of conflicting corporate interests as well as conflicting personal values? In a society in which special interests are fostered by corporate action, how do patients, who have no organization comparable to the American Medical Association, the American Nurses' Association, and the American Hospital Association, secure their interests?

Pellegrino forces us to consider the consequences of not recognizing the implications of a curing model for medicine. If one adopts a biomedical approach to medicine, does this imply that the issues of medical ethics will be determined by advances in medical science and technology? Does this imply that man is a biological or technical being with moral problems, as opposed to a moral being? Further, does beginning with a curative approach require an attempt to treat the whole person through so-called "holistic medicine"?

Pellegrino's contention that a caring approach to medical practice is humanistic, moral, and holistic by its nature suggests the need for philosophical considerations of the nature of caring. In other words, the conception of caring needs to be explored from a philosophical as well as from a medical context, as Pellegrino does in his essay.

Certainly, health care professionals will need to discuss how to combine Pellegrino's four senses of caring into integral care in actual medical practice. Also, ethicists will need to help the health care profession understand how the imperative for medical integral care is related to the general imperative to care for all human beings.

Pellegrino's treatment of a caring ethic, with its different modules and senses of the good, is a significant contribution to the substance and process of moral-medical decision making. But how do we get physicians to combine the morally good decision with the medically right decision? How do we get physicians, burdened by heavy case loads and the problem of keeping up with medical advances, to recognize the need for informal and formal considerations of such matters? How do we get medical schools to establish programs which will prepare medical students to wrestle with moral questions throughout their careers as physicians?

Gadow forces us to face the issue of whether caring and curing necessarily conflict. Do treatments by machines and professionals necessarily disrupt the dignity of the patient? Or, as she puts it, how can we use medical technology in attending to the "objectness" of the person without reducing the person to the moral status of an object?

Gadow contends that the nurse should be personally "related to" and involved with the patient. How can this be accomplished, when institutions require nurses to fulfill specific roles which encourage impersonal relationships between nurse and patient? If the nurse is to share personal views with the patient, how is she to do so without causing conflict with the physician or institution?

If touching is a way of overcoming a tendency to turn patients into objects, how is this to be done in a society in which sensuous and intimate touching is almost automatically associated with sexuality? How can touching occur spontaneously when professional models dictate that most direct care not be done by nurses and that new, technical equipment lessens the need to touch when one is carrying out nurses' functions? How can nurses learn that new technology can afford them more time and greater freedom to be with patients, rather than dictate their relationships to patients? How can those who set policy in hospitals and other health care institutions be persuaded that technological advances should be used to make nurses more available to patients?

Aroskar raises the question whether conflicts between physicians and nurses result from very different experiences of the world of work. This contention suggests that philosophers who use phenomenological techniques should assist physicians, nurses, and other health care workers and institutional personnel to understand each other's experience of the world of work.

Her suggestion that conflicts between physician and

nurse may result from male and female models for understanding moral issues raises two interesting questions. Do most physicians, being male, think more in terms of competing rights and reason from abstract moral principles, whereas most nurses, being female, think of moral issues in terms of conflicting responsibilities? How can a caring, relational ethic be appraised by its relevance and appropriateness for dealing with moral issues concerning health care, rather than by "gender designation"?

Aroskar asks us to consider the effect of regarding health services as commodities. Surely we need to consider the moral and medical implications of considering physicians and nurses as health care providers and patients as consumers. Certainly, in hospitals, the power of the physician would be enhanced by this interpretation, while that of the nurse will be lessened. After all, physicians bring patients to the hospital while nurses increase personnel costs. Since physicians and nurses claim the special privileges of professionals who serve the public, how can they work within a commercial framework without taking financial advantage of patients or compromising their professional standards?

Engelhardt contends that medicine and nursing have developed into a conglomerate of purposeful and accidental activities, motivated by altruistic, intellectual, and self-serving purposes. Therefore, both nursing and medicine consist of such varying activities that it is difficult to distinguish one from the other. His treatment suggests that both professions need to be considered in historical and contemporary contexts to determine what each should professionally, legally, and morally be entitled to do.

His contention that the domain of nurses consists of

what has been "left" to them by medicine suggests that nurses should continue to seek their own identity in relationship to others, but not dictated by others. Engelhardt's treatment also suggests the need to examine the legal privileges historically accorded to physicians in light of the changes in health care and society.

Engelhardt's contention that nurses are in between physicians' medical authority, supported by knowledge and legal and social authority, and patients, strengthened by increasing recognition of their rights, suggests several issues. Will nurses be able to find a conceptual core to define their place? Will their role continue to be defined by others, or will they determine their role and activities? If the latter, how will this be accomplished, given the power of physicians, patients, and health care institutions?

Engelhardt advocates that nurses and physicians work together in a partnership based on talent and skill, rather than professional designation, when this is possible within the constraints of law and social expectations. Will this co-partnership be better or worse for the patient? How will nurses acquire a co-partner status, given the historical limitation of their profession? And how will the new co-partnership between physician and nurse be related to the wishes of the patient or to the demands of the professions?

In short, with the changing relationships of physicians, nurses, and patients, how can conflicts resulting from differences in what the professionals wish, what the patients want, and what is best for the patients be adjudicated?

Zaner, directly examining their experiences of illness and hospitalization, helps us understand what patients want. His use of phenomenological methods suggests a way of studying the meaning of the experiences of all involved in health care. What does it mean to be a nurse, or a physician, from the perspective of the person who gives health care? What does it mean to experience illness as a patient? Can nurses and physicians understand their relationship to each other by examining their respective experience of each other in work relationships? How do health care workers come to understand the meaning of being ill and being a patient from the perspective of a patient?

While all conference leaders stress the importance of truth-telling, Zaner points out that truth-telling should take the form of communication between health care workers and patients concerning day-to-day treatment and care. In their treatment, patients often attempt to find clues concerning their prognosis. Lack of understanding often distorts the meaning of treatment, which creates unnecessary anxiety for the patient.

How can health care workers, often wrapped up in their day-to-day professional activities, learn to think from the patient's perspective? How can they help the patient deal with the existential crises which come from fearing debilitation or loss of life? What kind of education do they need to help patients face the existential questions of life and death, when their illness forces them to face their finiteness?

Zaner's contention that patients want to know that those who "care for them" really care raises the question of how we help health care workers recognize the difference between health care and health-care management. How can health care workers understand caring as a moral imperative and human way of being, as opposed to effective professional role-assuming or good hospital policy?

By pointing out that patients want professional care

Further Considerations

within the context of personal care, Zaner brings into focus the major consideration called for by the leaders of the conference. They all contend that caring, as a human way of being and as a moral imperative, should be the foundation of the relationship between physician, nurse, and patient. Further, they suggest that curing, with its stress on science and technology, should be incorporated and utilized within the caring relationship.

Thus, rather than adhering to the bioethical approach, they call on us to build health care relationships and medical ethics on the foundation of caring. Further, they give us valuable direction for accomplishing this formidable task.

Notes

CHAPTER 1 (PELLEGRINO)

1. Edmund Pellegrino, "The Sociocultural Impact of Twentieth-Century Therapeutics," in *The Therapeutic Revolution: Essays in the Social History of American Medicine*, ed. Morris J. Vogel and Charles E. Rosenberg (Philadelphia: University of Pennsylvania Press, 1979), pp. 245–66.

2. Donald Seldin, "The Medical Model: Biomedical Science as the Basis of Medicine," *Beyond Tomorrow* (New York: Rockefeller University Press, 1977).

3. George Engel, "The Clinical Application of the Biopsychosocial Model," *American Journal of Psychiatry*, 137:5:535–44.

4. Edmund Pellegrino and David Tomasma, *A Philosophical Basis for Medical Practice* (New York: Oxford University Press, 1981).

5. *Informed Consent: Current Opinions of the Judicial Council of the American Medical Association* (1981), p. 25.

6. Edmund D. Pellegrino, "Moral Choice, the Good of the Patient and the Patient's Good," paper delivered at Conference on Moral Choice and Medical Crisis, East Carolina University School of Medicine, Greenville, N.C., March 16–18, 1983. In press.

7. Leon Kass, "Professing Ethically," *Journal of the American Medical Association* 249 (1983): 1305–10; Edmund D. Pellegrino, "Toward a Reconstruction of Medical Morality: The Primacy of the Act of Profession and the Fact of Illness," *Journal of Medicine and Philosophy* 4 (March 1979): 32–56.

8. *Scribonii Largi Compositiones*, ed. Georgius, Helmreich, Lipsiae (1887); Ludwig Edelstein, "Professional Ethics of the Greek Physician," in *Ancient Medicine*, ed. Owsei Temkin and C. Lilian Temkin (Baltimore: Johns Hopkins Press, 1967), pp. 319–49.

9. Albert Camus, "Neither Victims or Executioners," *Continuum* (1980), p. 57.

10. Harvey Cushing, *Consecratio Medici and Other Papers* (Boston: Little, Brown, 1929), pp. 3–13.

Notes to Chapter 2

CHAPTER 2 (GADOW)

1. Shirley Steele and Vera Harmon, *Values Clarification in Nursing*, 2d ed. (Norwalk, Conn.: Appleton-Century-Crofts, 1983).

2. Robert A. Burt, *Taking Care of Strangers* (New York: Free Press, 1979), p. 167.

3. Paul Ramsey, "The Indignity of 'Death with Dignity,'" *Hastings Center Report* 2 (May 1974): 47–62; Dallas M. High, "Is 'Natural Death' an Illusion?" *Hastings Center Report* 8 (August 1978): 37–42.

4. Sally Gadow, "Touch and Technology: Two Paradigms of Patient Care," *Journal of Religion and Health* 23 (1): 67–68.

5. Richard Zaner, "Chance and Morality: The Dialysis Phenomenon," in *The Humanity of the Ill: Phenomenological Perspectives*, ed. Victor Kestenbaum (Knoxville: University of Tennessee Press, 1982), pp. 39–68.

6. Harold Bursztajn et al., *Medical Choices, Medical Chances* (New York: Delacorte, 1981).

7. J. Churchill, "Gods, Frogs, and Sojourns," *Soundings*, 65 (1982): 2.

8. Sally Gadow, "Basis for Nursing Ethics: Paternalism, Consumerism, or Advocacy?" *Hospital Progress* 64 (1983): 62–67.

9. Sally Gadow, "Existential Advocacy: Philosophical Foundation of Nursing," in *Nursing: Images and Ideals: Opening Dialogue with the Humanities*, ed. Stuart Spicker and Sally Gadow (New York: Springer, 1980), pp. 79–101.

10. Gadow, "Touch and Technology."

11. Edith Wyshcogrod, "Empathy and Sympathy as Tactile Encounter," *Journal of Medicine and Philosophy* 6 (1981): 25–43.

12. Richard Wilbur, "Advice to a Prophet," in *The Poems of Richard Wilbur* (New York: Harcourt Brace Jovanovich, 1963), p. 7.

13. W. H. Auden, "Surgical Ward," in *The Physician in Literature*, ed. Norman Cousins (Philadelphia: W. B. Saunders, 1982).

14. William F. May, "Who Cares for the Elderly?" *Hastings Center Report* 12 (1982): 31–37.

15. Ronald Blythe, *The View in Winter* (New York: Harcourt Brace Jovanovich, 1979), p. 82.

16. Martin Buber, *Between Man and Man* (New York: Macmillan, 1965), p. 19.

CHAPTER 3 (AROSKAR)

1. National Commission on Nursing, *Initial Report and Preliminary Recommendations* (Chicago: Hospital Research and Educational Trust, 1981), pp. 5, 10.

2. Timothy Sheard, "The Structure of Conflict in Nurse-Physician Relations," *Supervisor Nurse* 11 (August 1980): 14–15, 17–18.

3. Ibid., p. 18.

4. Carol Gilligan, *In a Different Voice: Psychological Theory and Women's Development* (Cambridge, Mass.: Harvard University Press, 1982), p. 19.

5. Lisa H. Newton, "To Whom Is the Nurse Accountable? A Philosophical Perspective," *Connecticut Medicine* 43 (October 1979): 7–9.

6. JoAnn Ashley, *Hospitals, Paternalism, and the Role of the Nurse* (New York: Teachers College Press, 1976), p. 17.

7. James L. Muyskens, *Moral Problems in Nursing: A Philosophical Investigation* (Totowa, N.J.: Rowman and Littlefield, 1982), pp. 41–42.

8. President's Commission for the Study of Ethical Problems in Medicine and Biomedical and Behavioral Research, *Making Health Care Decisions* (Washington, D.C.: U.S. Government Printing Office, October 1982), 1:3.

9. "Price Competitive Scheme Rocks Coast Hospitals," *American Journal of Nursing* 83 (February 1983): 196, 214, 216, 218.

10. Paul Starr, *The Social Transformation of American Medicine* (New York: Basic Books, 1982).

11. Edmund Erde, "Notions of Teams and Team Talk in

Notes to Chapter 4

Health Care," *Law, Medicine & Health Care* 9 (October 1981): 26–28.

CHAPTER 4 (ENGELHARDT)

1. See Lester King, "Some Basic Explanations of Disease: An Historian's Viewpoint," in *Evaluation and Explanation in the Biomedical Sciences*, eds. H. Tristram Engelhardt Jr. and Stuart F. Spicker (Dordrecht, Holland: D. Reidel Publishing Co., 1975), pp. 11–27.

2. The role of values in concepts of health and disease has been widely discussed. I take a weak normativist understanding of disease concepts in "The Concepts of Health and Disease," in *Evaluation and Explanation in the Biomedical Sciences* (pp. 125–41). See Also, H. Tristram Engelhardt Jr., "Ideology and Etiology," *Journal of Medicine and Philosophy* 1 (September 1976): 256–68; Joseph Margolis, "The Concept of Disease," *Journal of Medicine and Philosophy* 1 (1976): 238–55; and Lester King, "What Is Disease?" *Philosophy of Science* 21 (July 1954): 193–203.

Christopher Boorse has, on the contrary, argued for a value-neutral notion of the concepts of disease. See "On the Distinction between Disease and Illness," *Philosophy and Public Affairs* 5 (Fall 1975): 49–68; "What a Theory of Mental Health Should Be," *Journal for the Theory of Social Behavior* 6 (1976): 61–84; "Wright on Functions," *The Philosophical Review* 85 (January 1976): 70–86; "Health as a Theoretical Concept," *Philosophy of Science* 44 (December 1977): 542–73.

For a recent response of mine to Boorse, see "The Role of Values in the Discovery of Illness," in *Contemporary Issues in Bioethics* (2d ed.), ed. Tom Beauchamp and LeRoy Walters (Belmont, Calif.: Wadsworth, 1982), pp. 73–75.

3. Talcott Parsons, *The Social System* (New York: Free Press, 1951); "The Mental Hospital as a Type of Organization," in *The Patient and the Mental Hospital*, ed. Milton Greenblatt et al. (Glencoe, Ill.: Free Press, 1957), pp. 108–29; "Definitions of Health and Illness in the Light of American Values and Social

Structure," in *Patients, Physicians and Illness*, ed. E. Gartly Jaco (Glencoe, Ill.: Free Press, 1958), pp. 165–87.

4. Vern L. Bullough, "Licensure and the Medical Monopoly," in *The Law and the Expanding Nursing Role* (2d ed.), ed. Bonnie Bullough (New York: Appleton-Century-Crofts, 1980), pp. 14–22.

5. *McConnel v. Williams*, 361 Pa. 355, 65 A. 2nd 243 (1959).

6. Helen Creighton, ed., *Law Every Nurse Should Know*, 4th ed. (Philadelphia: W. B. Saunders, 1981).

7. A discussion of the difference between physician *assistant* and *associate* is provided in *The Physician's Assistant: Today and Tomorrow*, ed. Alfred M. Sadler Jr., Blair L. Sadler, and Ann A. Bliss (New Haven, Conn.: Yale University Press, 1972), along with other very helpful information comparing physician assistants and nurses. See also James F. Cawley and Archie S. Golden, "Nonphysicians in the United States: Manpower Policy in Primary Care," *Journal of Public Health Policy* 4 (March 1983): 76.

8. American Psychiatric Association, *Diagnostic and Statistical Manual of Mental Disorders*, 3d ed. (Washington, D.C.: American Psychiatric Association, 1980).

9. Alfred Schutz and Thomas Luckmann. *The Structures of the Life-World*, trans. Richard M. Zaner and H. Tristram Engelhardt Jr. (Evanston: Northwestern University Press, 1973).

10. For an excellent discussion of these issues, see Richard E. Flathman, "Power, Authority, and Rights in the Practice of Medicine," in *Responsibility in Health Care*, ed. George J. Agich (Dordrecht, Holland: D. Reidel Publishing Co., 1982), pp. 105–25.

11. H. Tristram Engelhardt Jr., "Bioethics in Pluralist Societies," *Perspectives in Biology and Medicine* 26 (Autumn 1982): 64–78.

12. *Natanson v. Kline*, 186 Kan. 393, 350 P. 2d 1093, 1104 (1960).

13. *Canterbury v. Spence*, 464 F. 2d 772 (D.C. Cir. 1972).

14. *Olmstead v. United States*, 277 U.S. 438, 478 (1928) (Brandeis, J., dissenting).

15. *In re President and Directors of Georgetown College, Inc.* 331 F. 2d 1000, 1017 (D.C. Cir.), *cert denied*, 337 U.S. 978 (1964).

16. *Tuma* v. *Board of Nursing* 593 P. 2d 711 (S. Ct. Idaho 1979).

17. One might consider here *Nursing: Concepts of Practice,* by Dorthea E. Orem, 2d ed. (New York: McGraw-Hill, 1980).

18. William L. Prosser, *Law of Torts,* 4th ed. (St. Paul, Minn.: West Publishing Co., 1983), pp. 36–37. "The gist of the action for battery is not the hostile intent of the defendant, but rather the absence of consent to the contact on the part of the plaintiff. The defendant may be liable where he has intended only a joke, or even a compliment, as where an unappreciative woman is kissed without her consent, or a misguided effort is made to render assistance. The plaintiff is entitled to protection according to the usages of decent society, and hostile contacts, or those which are contrary to all good manners, need not be tolerated."

19. *Schloendorff* v. *Society of New York Hospital,* 211 N.Y. 125, 105 N.E. 92, 93 (1914).

20. *Griswold* v. *Connecticut,* 381 U.S. 479 (1965).

21. *Roe* v. *Wade,* 410 U.S. 113, 93 S.G. 707, 35 L. Ed. 2d 147 (1973).

CHAPTER 5 (ZANER)

1. Richard M. Zaner, "Chance and Morality: The Dialysis Phenomenon," in *The Humanity of the Ill,* ed. Victor Kestenbaum (Knoxville: University of Tennessee Press, 1982), pp. 37–68.

2. Lee Foster, "Man and Machine: Life without Kidneys," *Hastings Center Report* 6 (June 1976): 6–8.

3. Mary Rawlinson, "Medicine's Discourse and the Practice of Medicine," in *The Humanity of the Ill,* ed. Victor Kestenbaum (Knoxville: University of Tennessee Press, 1982), pp. 69–85.

4. Edmund D. Pellegrino, "Being Ill and Being Healed: Some Reflections on the Grounding of Medical Morality," in *The Humanity of the Ill,* ed. Victor Kestenbaum (Knoxville: University of Tennessee Press, 1982), pp. 157–66.

5. Robert C. Hardy, *Sick: How People Feel about Being Sick and What They Think of Those Who Care for Them* (Chicago: Teach'em, Inc., 1978).

6. Alfred Schutz, "The Stranger," in Alfred Schutz, *Collected*

Papers, vol. II: *Studies in Social Theory,* ed. Arvid Brodersen (*Phaenomenologica* 15) (The Hague: Martinus Nijhoff, 1964), pp. 91–104.

7. Robert C. Hardy, "My Turn," unpublished reflections on his book *Sick* (see above).

8. Ibid.

9. Cited in Herbert Spiegelberg, "Good Fortune Obligates: Albert Schweitzer's Second Ethical Principle," *Ethics* 85 (1975): 234.

10. Foster, "Man and Machine," pp. 6–8.

11. Quoted in Spiegelberg, "Good Fortune Obligates," p. 234.

Selected Bibliography

NURSE-PATIENT RELATIONSHIPS

Aroskar, Mila. "Ethics of Nurse-Patient Relationships," *Nurse Educator* VI (March–April 1980): 18–20.

Aroskar, Mila A. "The Fractured Image: The Public Stereotype of Nursing and the Nurse." In *Nursing: Images and Ideals,* ed. Stuart Spicker and Sally Gadow. New York: Springer Publishing Co., 1980.

Brook, Dan. "The Nurse-Patient Relation: Some Rights and Duties." In *Nursing: Images and Ideals,* ed. Stuart Spicker and Sally Gadow. New York: Springer Publishing Co., 1980.

Gadow, Sally. "Existential Advocacy: Philosophical Foundation of Nursing." In *Nursing: Images and Ideals,* ed. Stuart Spicker and Sally Gadow. New York: Springer Publishing Co., 1980.

Smith, Sherri. "Three Models of Nurse-Patient Relationship." in *Nursing: Images and Ideals,* ed. Stuart Spicker and Sally Gadow. New York: Springer Publishing Co., 1980.

NURSE-PHYSICIAN RELATIONSHIPS

Aroskar, Mila A. "When Doctor and Nurse Disagree: An Interface of Politics and Ethics" In *Troubling Problems in Medical Ethics,* ed. Marc D. Basson, Rachel Lipson, and Doreen Ganos, pp. 187–92. New York: Alan R. Liss, 1981.

Bell, Nora K. "Whose Autonomy Is at Stake? *Tuma* vs. *Board of Nursing.*" *American Journal of Nursing* 81 (June 1981): 1170–72.

Hull, Richard T. "Models of Nurse/Patient/Physician Relations." *Kansas Nurse* 55 (October 1980): 19–24.

MacElveen-Hoehn, Patricia. "The Cooperation Model for Care in Health and Illness." In *The Nursing Profession: A Time to Speak,* ed. Norma L. Chaska, pp. 515–39. New York: McGraw-Hill, 1983.

Selected Bibliography

PHYSICIAN-PATIENT RELATIONSHIPS

Berger, Michael, and Tristram Engelhardt. "Observation of a Physician-Patient," *Southern Medical Journal* 70 (August 1977): 988–90.

Engelhardt, Tristram. "The Patient as Person—An Empty Phrase?" *Texas Medicine* 71 (September 1975): 57–63.

———. "A Demand to Die" (a commentary on a case history). *Hastings Center Report* 5 (June 1975): 10, 47.

———. "Human Well-Being and Medicine: Some Basic Value Judgments in the Biomedical Sciences." In *Science, Ethics and Medicine*, ed. H. Tristram Engelhardt Jr. and Daniel Callahan, pp. 120–39. Hastings-on-Hudson, N.Y.: Hastings Center, 1976.

———. "Concept of Health." *Encyclopaedia Britannica 1977 Medical and Health Annual*, pp. 100–08.

———. "Some Persons Are Humans, Some Humans Are Persons, and the World Is What the Humans Make of It." In *Philosophical Medical Ethics: Its Nature and Significance*, ed. Stuart F. Spicker and H. Tristram Engelhardt Jr., pp. 183–94. Dordrecht, Holland: Reidel Publishing Co., 1977.

———. "Medicine and the Concept of Person." in *Ethical Issues in Death and Dying*, ed. Tom L. Beauchamp and Seymour Perlin, pp. 271–84. Engelwood Cliffs, N.J.: Prentice-Hall, 1978.

———. "To Treat or Not to Treat: The Dilemma" (by H. Tristram Engelhardt Jr. et al.). *Heart and Lung* 7 (May/June 1979): 499–504.

———. "Rights to Health Care: A Critical Appraisal." *Journal of Medicine and Philosophy* 4 (June 1979): 113–17.

———. "Ethical Issues in Pain Management." In *Pain and Society*, ed. H. W. Kosterlitz and Lars Y. Terenius, pp. 461–80. Weinheim, West Germany: Chemie, 1980.

———. "Value Imperialism and Exploitation in Sex Therapy." In *Ethical Issues in Sex Therapy and Research*, vol. II, ed. William H. Masters, Virginia E. Johnson, and Robert C. Kolodny, pp. 109–37. Boston: Little, Brown, 1980.

———. "The Rule of Values in the Discovery of Illness." In

Selected Bibliography

Contemporary Issues in Bioethics (2d ed.), ed. Tom Beauchamp and Leroy Walter, pp. 73–75. Belmont, Calif.: Wadsworth, 1982.

Hull, Richard. "Ethics: Models of Nurse/Patient/Physician Relationships." *Kansas Nurse* (October 1980).

Pellegrino, Edmund D. "Physicians, Patients and Society: Some New Tensions in Medical Ethics." In *Human Aspects of Biomedical Innovation*, ed. Everett Mendelson, Judith P. Swazey, and Irene Tavis, pp. 77–97 and 219–20. Cambridge, Mass.: Harvard University Press, 1971.

————. "The Changing Matrix of Clinical Decision Making in the Hospital." In *Organization Research on Health Institutions*, ed. Basil S. Georgopoulis, pp. 302–28. Ann Arbor: University of Michigan Press, 1972.

————. "The Right to Die: Should a Doctor Decide?" *U.S. News & World Report*, November 3, 1975, p. 53.

————. "Protection of Patients' Rights and the Doctor-Patient Relationship." *Preventive Medicine* 4 (December 1975): 398–403.

————. "Profession, Patient, Compassion, Consent: Meditations on Medical Philosophy." *Connecticut Medicine* 42 (March 1978): 175–78.

————. "Ethics and the Moment of Clinical Truth" (editorial). *Journal of the American Medical Association* 239 (March 6, 1978): 960–61.

————. "Protection of Patients' Rights and the Doctor-Patient Relationship." In *Matters of Life and Death: Crises in Biomedical Ethics*, ed. John C. Thomas, pp. 307–15. Toronto: Samuel Stevens Publisher, 1978.

————. "The Physician-Patient Relationship in Preventive Medicine: Reply to Robert Dickman." *Journal of Medicine and Philosophy* 5 (September 1980): 208–12.

————. "Philosophy of Medicine as the Source of Medical Ethics." In *Metamedicine*, ed. David C. Thomasma, 2: 5–11. Dordrecht: Reidel, 1981.

————. "The Moral Foundations for Valid Consent." Proceedings of American Cancer Society, Third National Conference on Human Values and Cancer, Washington, D.C., April 23–

25, 1981. New York: American Cancer Society, pp. 171–78.

Zaner, Richard. *The Context of Self: A Phenomenological Inquiry Using Medicine as a Clue.* Athens: Ohio University Press, 1981.

———. "Ethics and Dialysis." In *Psychological Factors in Hemodialysis and Transplantation* (Transactions of First International Conference), ed. Norman B. Levy.

———. "The Unanchored Leaf: Humanities and the Discipline of Care." *Texas Reports on Biology and Medicine* 32 (Spring 1974): 29–43.

———. "The Cutting Edge in Medical Ethics." *Southwest Review* 64 (Spring 1979): 131–38.

Contributors

Mila Ann Aroskar is associate professor, Public Health Nursing Program, School of Public Health, University of Minnesota. She is co-author of *Ethical Dilemmas and Nursing Practice*, which is in its second edition. She has written numerous articles, developed educational materials, and conducted research on ethical decision making in intensive care units.

Anne H. Bishop is professor of nursing, Lynchburg College. In 1976 she was named Outstanding Nurse of the Year by the Virginia Nurses' Association and from 1981 to 1983 was president of the Virginia League for Nursing. She has a longstanding interest in the ethics in nursing.

H. Tristram Engelhardt, Jr. is a professor in the Departments of Medicine and Community Medicine, Baylor College of Medicine, and a member of the Center for Ethics, Medicine and Social Issues. He was formerly the Rosemary Kennedy Professor of the Philosophy of Medicine at the Center for Bioethics, Kennedy Institute of Ethics, Georgetown University. An educator and a physician, he holds a Ph.D. in philosophy (as well as his M.D.). Among his numerous publications are *Mind-Body: A Categorical Relation, Bioethics: An Introduction and Critique,* and *Diseases and Healths: The Role of Values in Medical Explanations.*

Sally A. Gadow is an associate professor in the Institute for the Medical Humanities, University of Texas Medical Branch, and holds a Ph.D. in philosophy as well as an advanced degree in nursing. She has written numerous articles and chapters concerning philosophy and nursing, in addition to co-editing the well-known book, *Nursing, Images and Ideals: Opening Dialogue with the Humanities.*

Edmund D. Pellegrino is director of the Kennedy Institute for Ethics, as well as the John Carroll Professor of Medicine and Medi-

Contributors

cal Humanities at Georgetown University. He is former president of the Catholic University of America and the Yale–New Haven Medical Center, chancellor and vice-president for Health Affairs at the University of Tennessee, and was the founding chief executive of the Health Science Center of the State University of New York at Stony Brook. He is the author of over 250 publications on medical education and philosophy.

John R. Scudder, Jr. is professor of philosophy, Lynchburg College. He is author of *History of Disciple Theories of Religious Education* and co-author of *Meaning, Dialogue, and Enculturation: A Phenomenological Philosophy of Education* (forthcoming). He is a past president of the South Atlantic Philosophy of Education Society.

Richard M. Zaner, the Ann Geddes Stahlman professor of medical and clinical ethics at Vanderbilt University, has held a joint appointment in philosophy and medicine at Stony Brook University and the Easterwood Chair in philosophy at Southern Methodist University. An authority on the self and medicine, he is the author of three books, including *The Way of Phenomenology* and *The Context of Self: A Phenomenological Inquiry Using Medicine as a Clue.* He has written numerous articles and chapters, as well as edited books, on medicine and philosophy.

Index